Image-Based Case Studies in ENT AND HEAD & NECK SURGERY

Image-Based Case Studies in ENT AND HEAD & NECK SURGERY

Rahmat Omar MBBS (Malaya) MS ORL (UM)
Consultant Otolaryngologist and
Head and Neck Surgeon
Department of Otorhinolaryngology
Faculty of Medicine
University of Malaya, Kuala Lumpur, Malaysia

Prepageran Narayanan
MBBS (Malaya) MS ORL (UM) FRCS (Ed) FRCS (Glas)
Professor
Senior Consultant Otolaryngologist and
Head and Neck Surgeon
Department of Otorhinolaryngology
Faculty of Medicine
University of Malaya
Kuala Lumpur, Malaysia

Foreword
Ghauth Jasmon

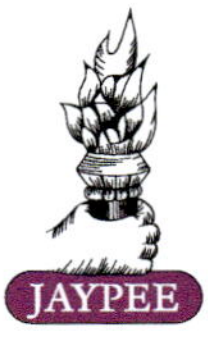

JAYPEE BROTHERS MEDICAL PUBLISHERS (P) LTD
New Delhi • Panama City • London • Dhaka • Kathmandu

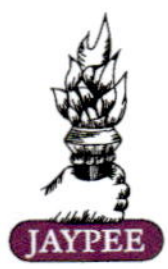

Jaypee Brothers Medical Publishers (P) Ltd.

Headquarters
EMCA House
23/23-B, Ansari Road, Daryaganj
New Delhi 110 002, India
Landline: +91-11-23272143, +91-11-23272703
+91-11-23282021, +91-11-23245672
E-mail: jaypee@jaypeebrothers.com

Corporate Office
Jaypee Brothers Medical Publishers (P) Ltd.
4838/24, Ansari Road, Daryaganj
New Delhi 110 002, India
Phone: +91-11-43574357
Fax: +91-11-43574314
E-mail: jaypee@jaypeebrothers.com

Overseas Office
JP Medical Ltd.
83, Victoria Street, London
SW1H 0HW (UK)
Phone: +44-20 3170 8910
E-mail: info@jpmedpub.com

EU GPSR Authorised Representative
Logos Europe, 9 rue Nicolas Poussin
17000, La Rochelle, France
Phone: +33 (0) 6 67 93 73 78
E-mail: Contact@logoseurope.eu

Website: www.jaypeebrothers.com
Website: www.jaypeedigital.com

Inquiries for bulk sales may be solicited at: jaypee@jaypeebrothers.com

Image-Based Case Studies in ENT and Head & Neck Surgery

First Edition: **2013,** Reprint 2025

ISBN 978-93-5090-089-5

Printed in India

Dedicated to

My beloved parents:
for your everlasting inspirations and motivations.
My family: Dr Salmah Ismail, Nur Rabbaniyyah, Muhammad Iqbal,
Ahmad Farhan, and Mursyid Syaqeer.
My students, past and present.

Rahmat Omar

The Divine Mother and My Family

Prepageran Narayanan

Foreword

It gives me a great pleasure to write a few words on the *Image-Based Case Studies in ENT and Head & Neck Surgery*.

I understand that this is the second book of this nature published by the authors; the successor of the first book which was an outstanding success. This proves that there is a demand for clear precise pictorial reference books as it enables the readers to appreciate the varied clinical presentations and its subsequent management in day-to-day clinical practice. This questions and answers book will complement the previous book which was an atlas. It is said a picture paints a thousand words and this is indeed true in clinical settings. This book covers the varied clinical images in different segments of otorhinolaryngology (ENT), ranging from otology, rhinology, head and neck and laryngology. It is a testament to the dedication and enthusiasm of the authors. I wish to congratulate the authors Associate Professor Dr Rahmat Omar and Professor Dr Prepageran on the publication of this book.

University of Malaya is committed to become a center of excellence in academic pursuit not only in Malaysia but also in the region and internationally. We encourage knowledge expansion and dissemination, and books written by young upcoming academicians are very much an integral part of the University of Malaya's effort to promote academics and culture of publishing among its academic staffs. I hope this will encourage more authors to put their wisdom and knowledge gathered over the years into books of similar nature to keep the readers updated and refreshed with core as well as current best practice information.

Finally, I would like to compliment the authors again and believe this book will be well accepted among a wide spectrum of readers ranging from medical students, primary care physicians to ENT masters students.

Ghauth Jasmon
Vice Chancellor
University of Malaya
50603 Kuala Lumpur

Preface

It is our pleasure to write a questions and answers book in ENT and Head and Neck Surgery which seems appropriate for the purpose of exercise and quick revision especially to our undergraduate and postgraduate students. The fundamental will still be the core of this book with applied and functional knowledge added for integration. These are based on real scenarios and clinical findings which were encountered during daily outpatient practice and in the operating table during surgery. The cases were carefully selected to represent the main issue of particular question.

Almost all the images were taken and edited by the first author. The book is divided into four sections; Otology, Rhinology, Head and Neck, and Laryngology. Special techniques like endoscopy and videostroboscopy were used to enable excellent high quality color photographs to be taken especially from the ear, nasal cavity, and larynx.

This book is complementary to the Ear Nose Throat Colour Atlas and Synopsis which was published earlier by University of Malaya Press. It would be an ideal resource for exam preparation and revision; hopefully readers would find it useful and practical. For qualified specialists and ENT surgeons, this book would be an indispensable quick reference.

We would like to thank the patients appearing in this book, as without their willingness and cooperation this work would not have been completed. Special thanks to the medical officers in training and colleagues from the Department of Otorhinolaryngology, University of Malaya, who had directly or indirectly contributed in any way in the production of this book.

Rahmat Omar
Prepageran Narayanan

Contents

Abbreviations

AA	:	atticoantral
BCC	:	basal cell carcinoma
BERA	:	brainstem evoked response audiometry
CA	:	carcinoma
CaHA	:	calcium hydroxyapatite
CAT	:	combined approach tympanoplasty
CO_2 laser	:	carbon dioxide laser
CP	:	cerebellopontine angle
CSF	:	cerebrospinal fluid
CSOM (AA)	:	chronic suppurative otitis media (atticoantral)
CSOM (TT)	:	chronic suppurative otitis media (tubotympanic)
CT scan	:	computed tomography-scan
DCR	:	dacryocystorhinostomy
DNS	:	deviated nasal septum
ET	:	Eustachian tube
FBC	:	full blood count
FNAC	:	fine needle aspiration cytology
FOR	:	fossa of Rosenmüller
GA	:	general anesthesia
HPE	:	histopathological examination
HRCT	:	high resolution computed tomography
IAM	:	internal auditory meatus
LPR	:	laryngopharyngeal reflux
MEE	:	middle ear effusion
MRI	:	magnetic resonance imaging
MRM	:	modified radical mastoidectomy
M&G	:	myringotomy and grommet
OMC	:	osteomeatal complex
PNS	:	postnasal space
PTA	:	pure tone audiogram
SNHL	:	sensorineural hearing loss
TB	:	tuberculosis
TM	:	tympanic membrane
TT	:	tubotympanic
VS	:	vestibular schwannoma

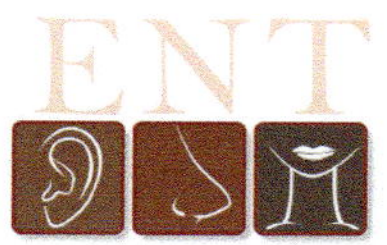

1 OTOLOGY

Questions

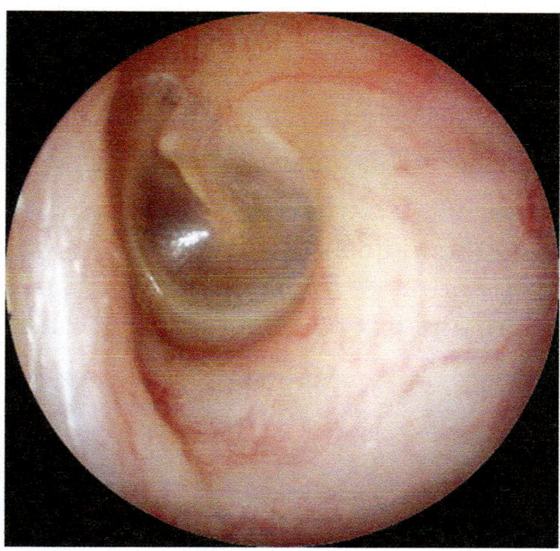

Q. 1. What does this picture show?

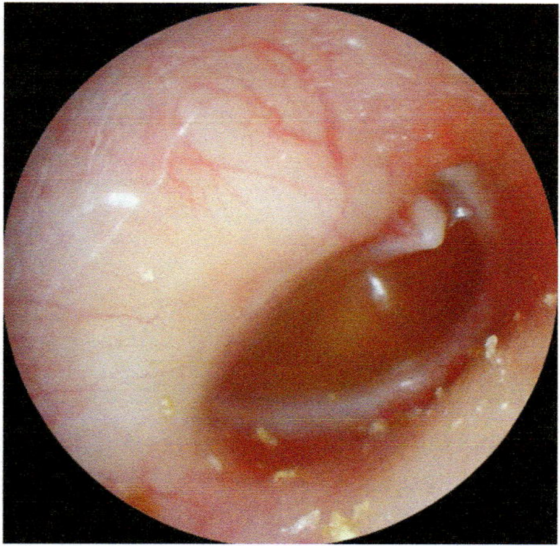

Q. 2. a. What does this otoendoscopic examination show?
b. Why does this occur?
c. What are the possible causes?

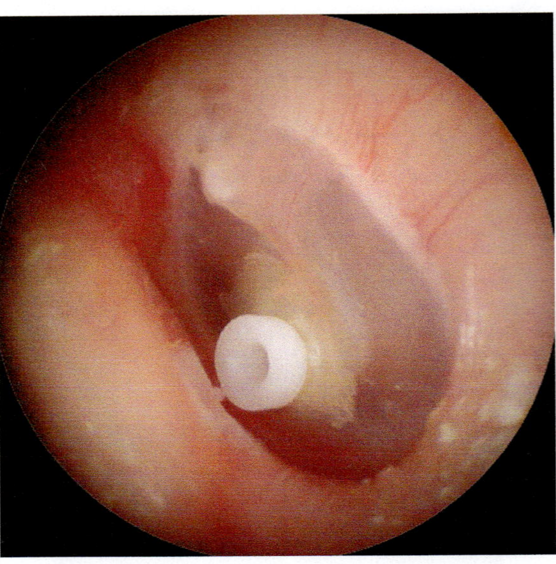

Q. 3. a. What procedure was taken as demonstrated in this picture?
b. What are the indications?
c. What are the considerations when performing the procedure and its potential complications?

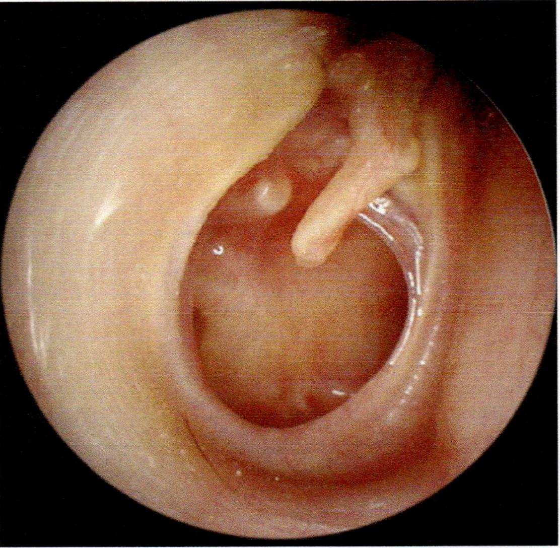

Q. 4. A middle-aged lady presented with reduced hearing affecting the right ear associated with the past history of recurrent ear discharge since childhood. Otoendoscopic examination and tuning fork test was performed.
a. Describe the findings.
b. What would be the expected tuning fork test result?
c. How this patient would be managed further?

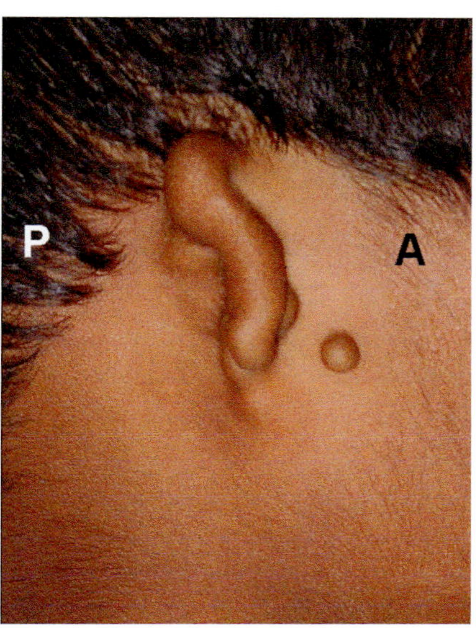

Q. 5. This is an image of the right ear.

a. What does it show?

b. What is the management?

(Abbreviations: A, anterior; P, posterior)

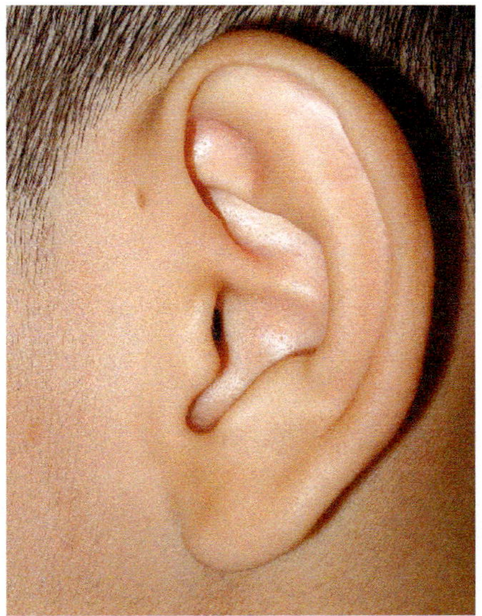

Q. 6. a. What is the abnormality seen?

b. What are the possible complications and the subsequent management?

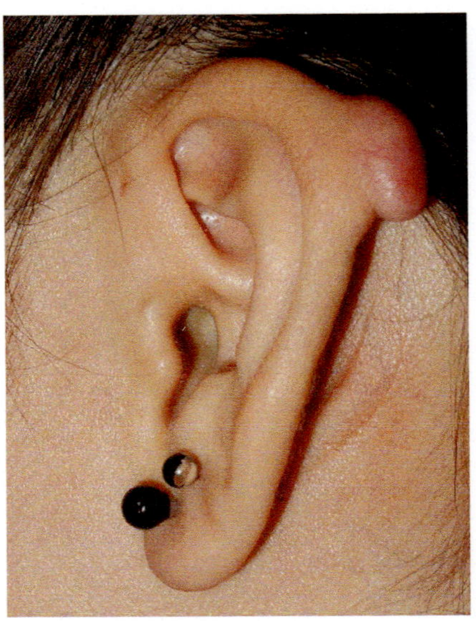

Q. 7. a. What is the diagnosis?
b. Explain the underlying pathology and the subsequent management.

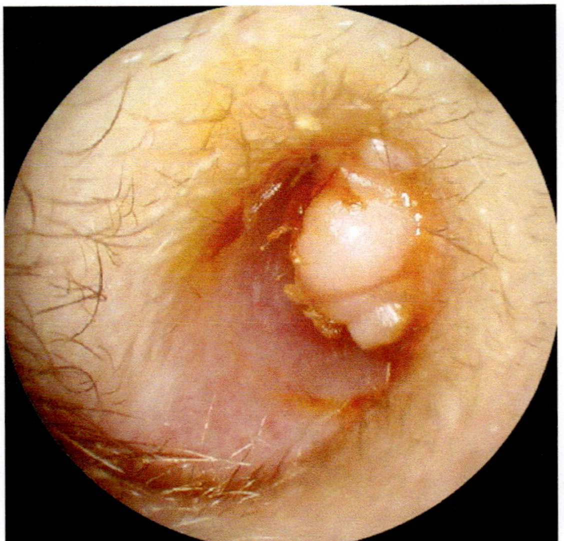

Q. 8. a. What does this picture show?
b. How would this patient be managed further?

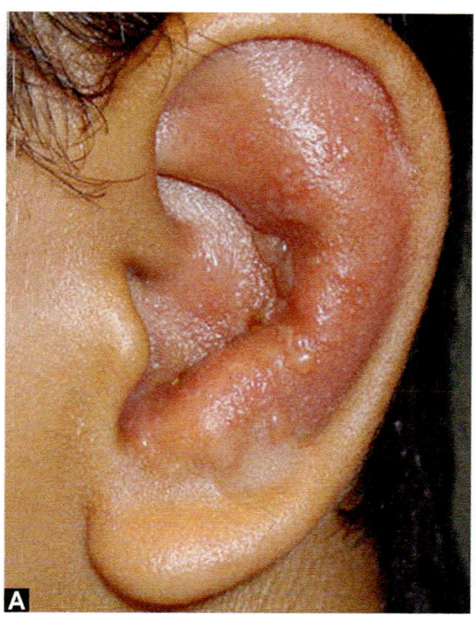

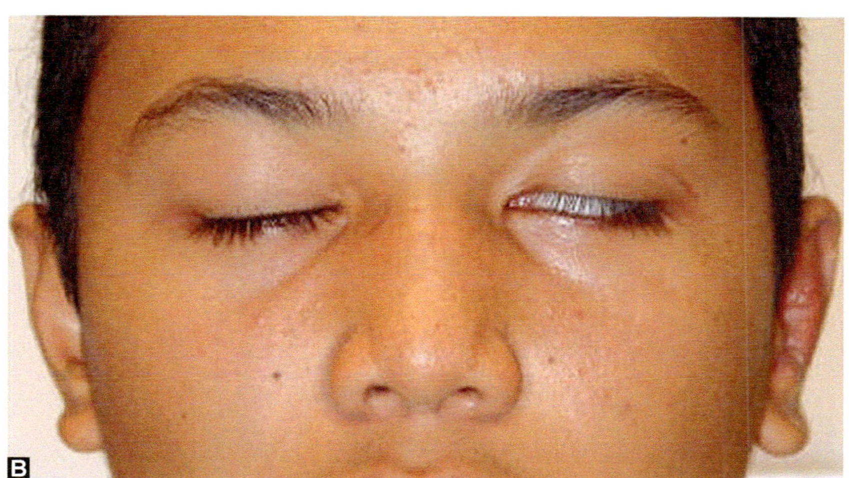

Q. 9. A male teenager presented with a painful left ear for 2 days duration followed by itchiness and inability to close the eye on the same side.

a. Describe the findings as shown.
b. What is the diagnosis?
c. Outline further management of this patient.

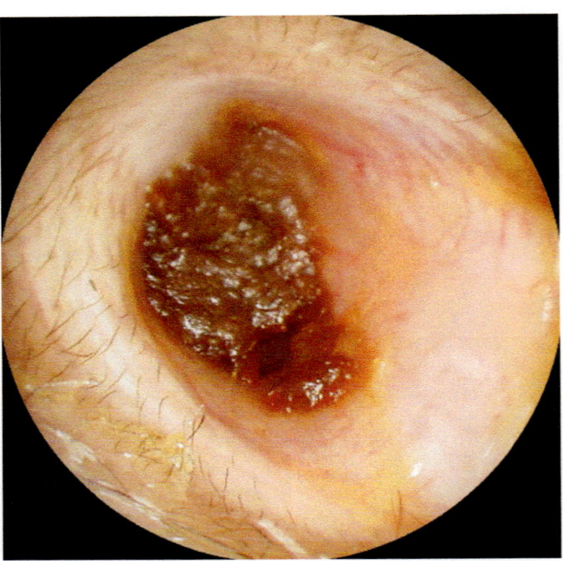

Q. 10. This is an otoendoscopic view of a patient who presented with the history of reduced hearing.

a. What is the diagnosis?

b. What are the other common clinical features?

c. How would this child be managed further?

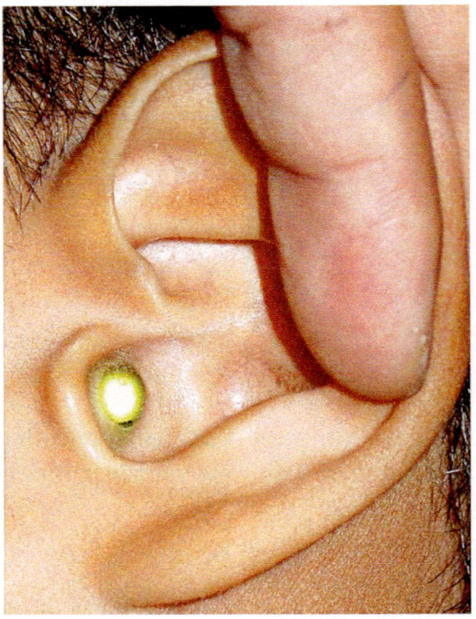

Q. 11. a. What does this examination of a child's ear show?

b. How is this condition managed?

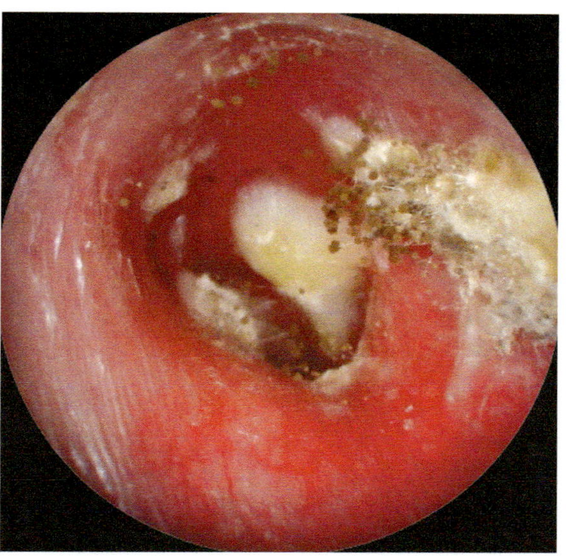

Q. 12. This patient presented with an itchy painful ear.
What is the diagnosis, etiology and the subsequent treatment?

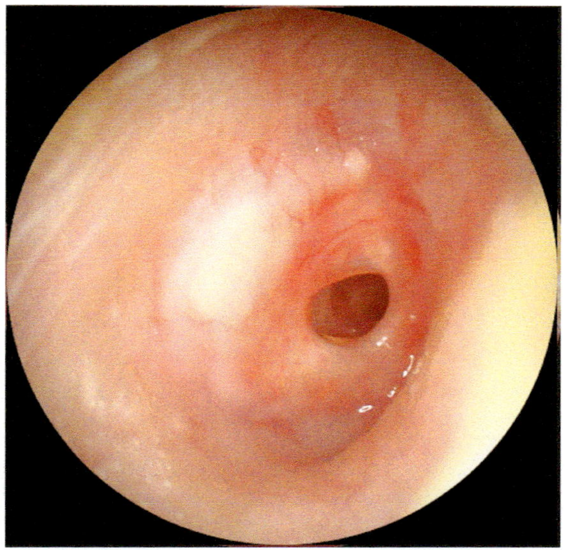

Q. 13. This patient presented with recurrent ear discharge.
What is the diagnosis, immediate and long-term management?

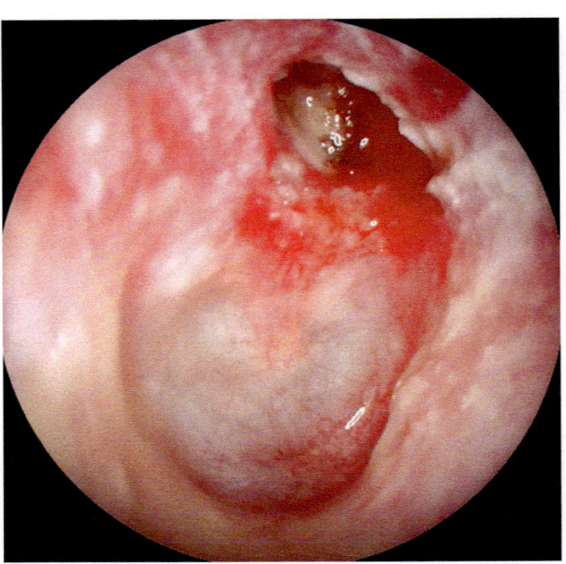

Q. 14. This patient presented with prolonged ear discharge. Otoscopic findings were as shown.

a. What is the diagnosis?

b. How is the presentation different from chronic suppurative otitis media (tubotympanic)?

c. How would this condition be managed further?

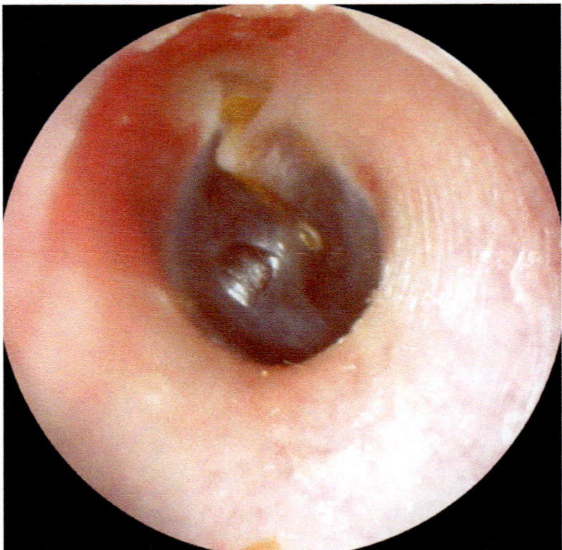

Q. 15. a. What does this otoscopy picture show?

b. What are the possible causes?

c. How is this condition managed?

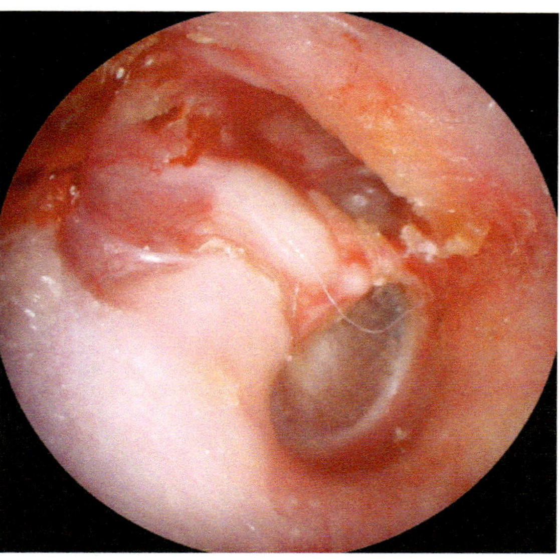

Q. 16. a. What does this picture reveal and what operation has been performed?
b. What are the potential complications related to the surgery?
c. What are the alternative procedures that can be carried out and in what condition?

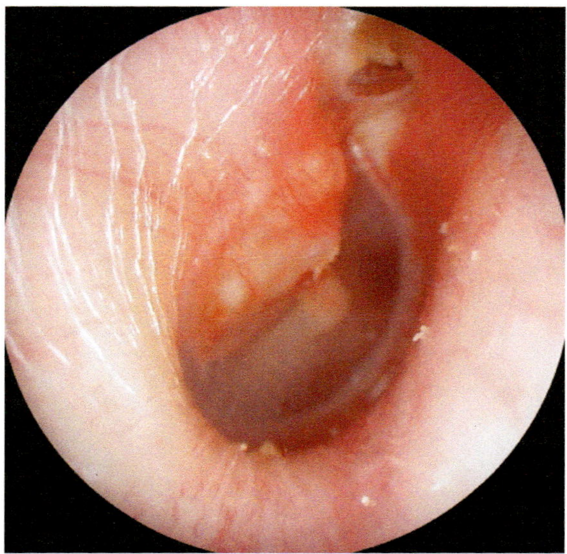

Q. 17. A 25-year-old gentleman presented with hearing loss as the only symptom. What is the diagnosis and its subsequent management?

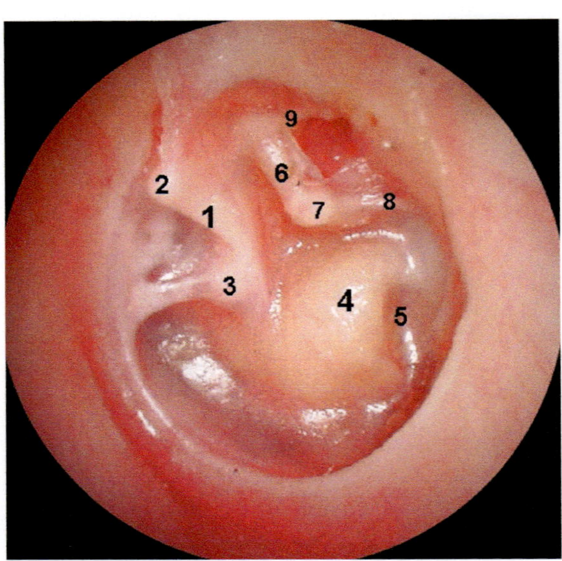

Q. 18. This is an otoscopic finding of a patient who presents with fullness of ear and mild hearing loss.

a. What does the otoendoscopy reveal?
b. Why is the hearing loss minimal?
c. What can we do further?

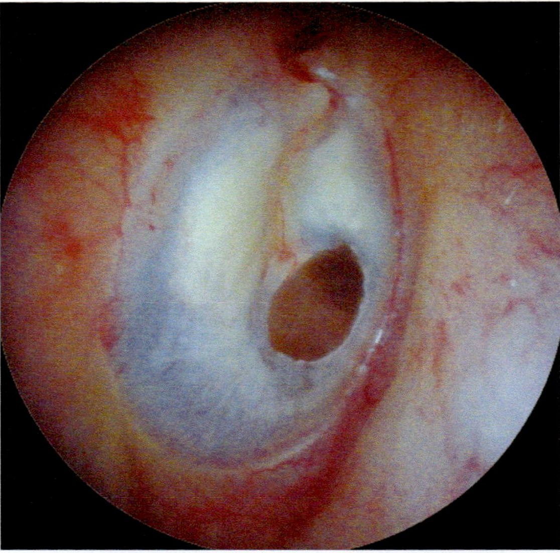

Q. 19. What is the pathology seen and what would be the next course of action in this patient with hearing loss?

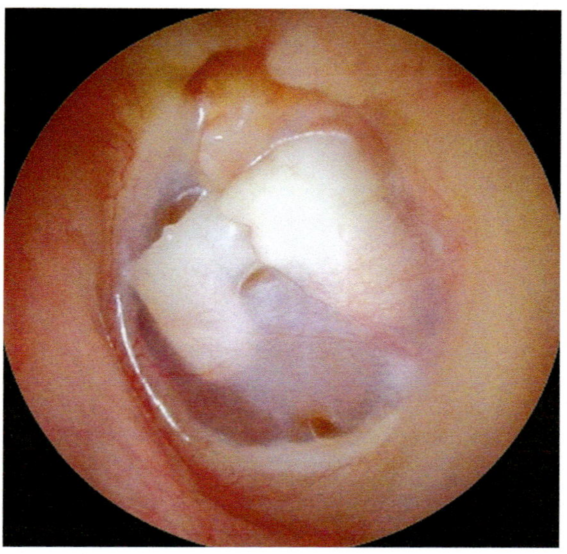

Q. 20. a. What does this picture show?
b. What would have contributed to this appearance?

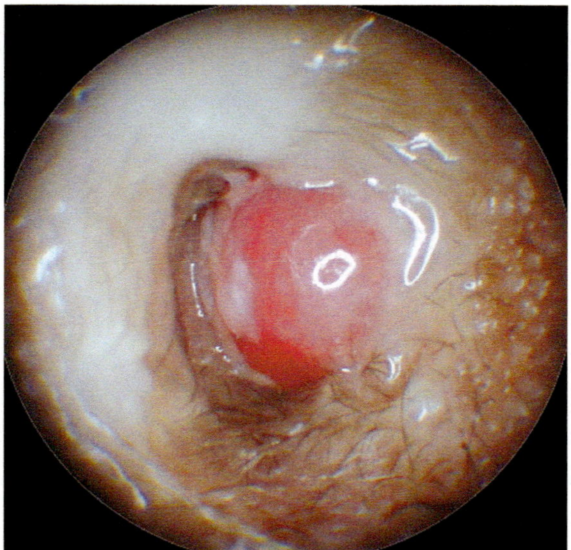

Q. 21. This is the image of an ear canal.
a. What does this picture show?
b. How would this condition be managed further?

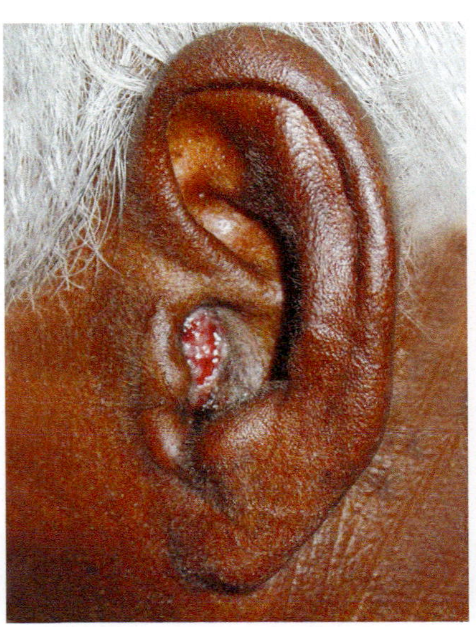

Q. 22. This patient presented with bleeding from the left ear.
  a. What are the possible diagnoses?
  b. Outline the subsequent management.

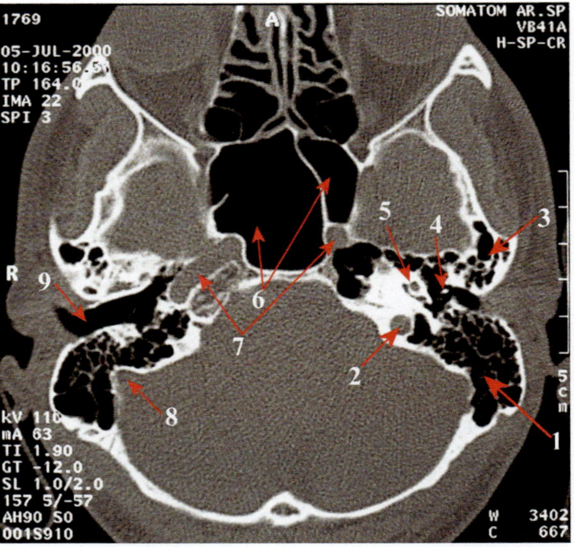

Q. 23. a. What is this image?
  b. Name the parts that are numbered.

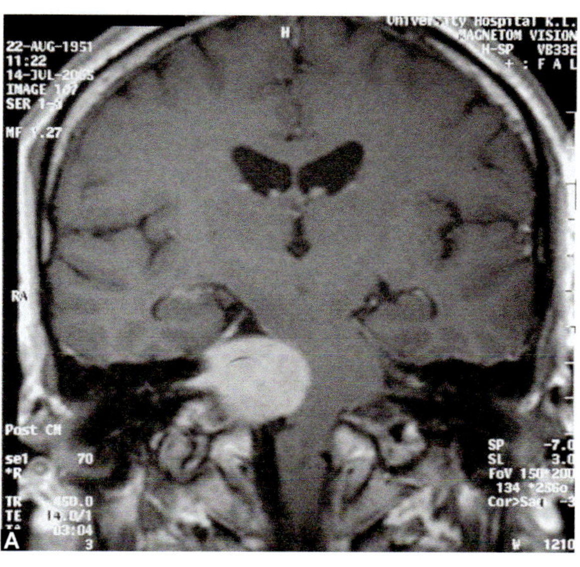

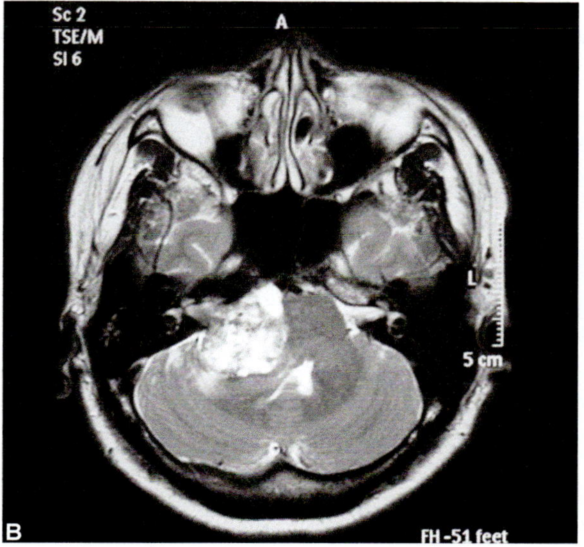

Q. 24. a. What does this image show?

b. What are the differential diagnoses and how do you differentiate them?

c. What are the clinical features?

d. Outline the subsequent management.

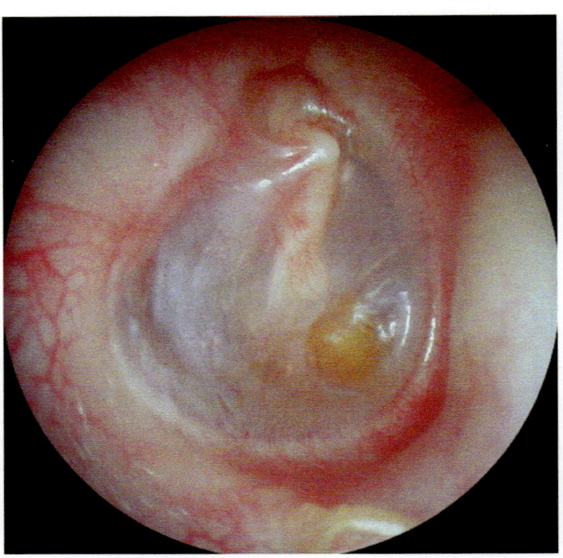

Q. 25. This is an otoendoscopic view of a middle-aged female who complains of an ear blockage.
What do you see and the probable underlying pathology?

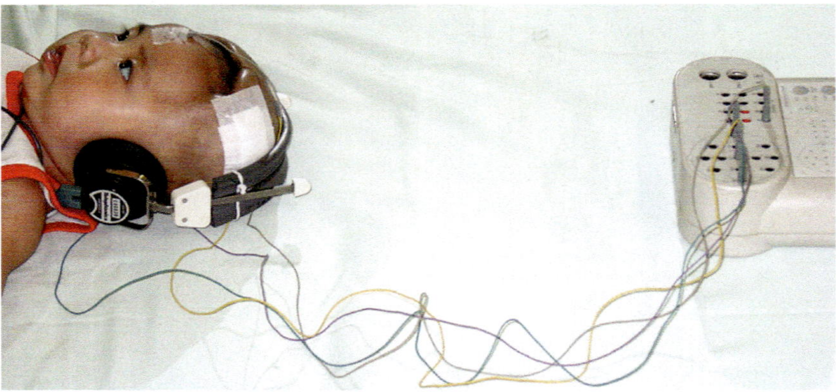

Q. 26. This child is undergoing a hearing assessment.
What is the name of the test and its indications?

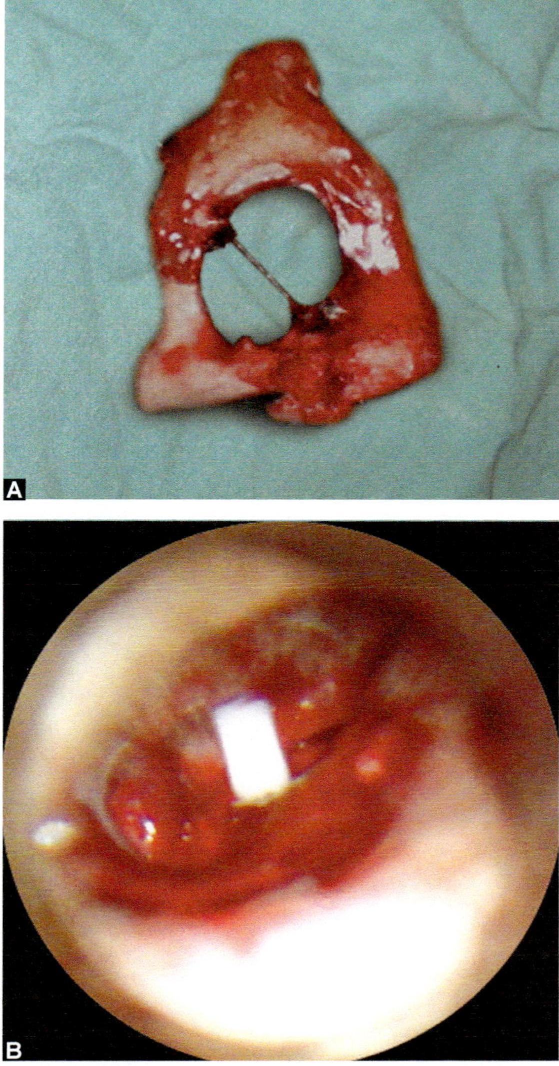

Q. 27. A 45-year-old lady complained of right-sided hearing loss, which has become worse since her last pregnancy. Examination revealed a normal tympanic membrane and the tuning fork tests showed a moderately severe conductive hearing loss. She underwent surgery and reconstructive procedure was performed.

a. What is the diagnosis?
b. Describe the findings as shown in Figures (A) and (B)?
c. What procedure would probably have been performed?

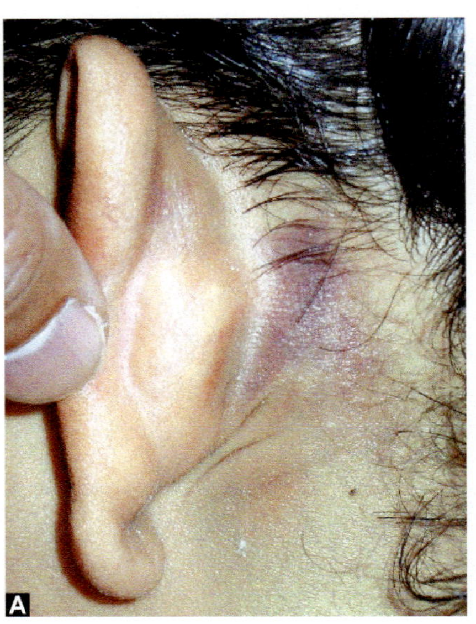

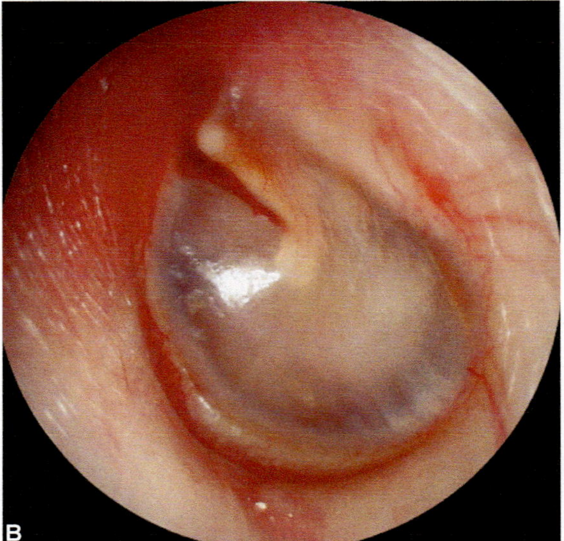

Q. 28. A 29-year-old lady was involved in a road traffic accident and sustained intracranial injury. She was referred to the ENT team few days later for the complaint of reduced hearing affecting the left side. Otological examination revealed above findings.

a. What is the clinical sign demonstrated in Figure (A) and on otoscopic evaluation in Figure (B)?
b. What other signs should be looked for?
c. How would this patient be managed further?

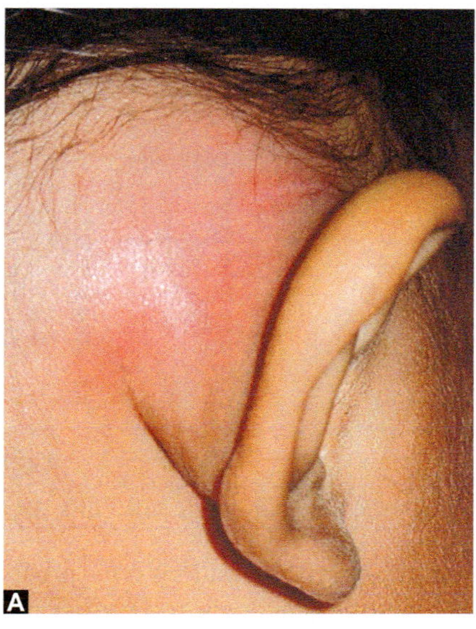

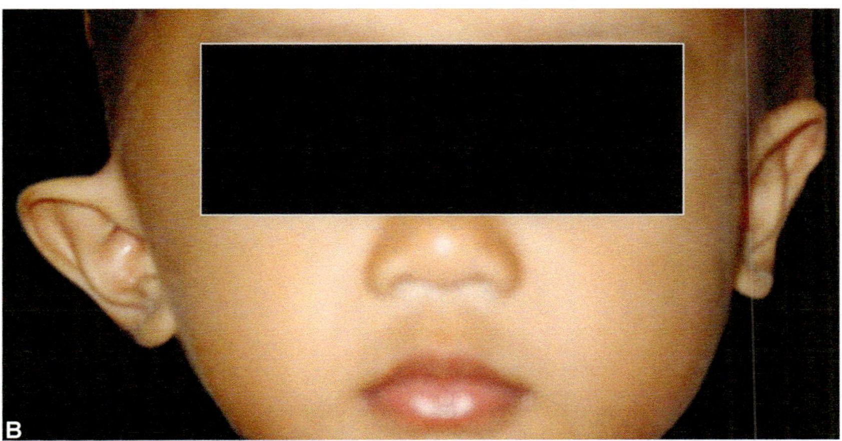

Q. 29. This child presented in the clinic with the above findings. What is your diagnosis and subsequent management?

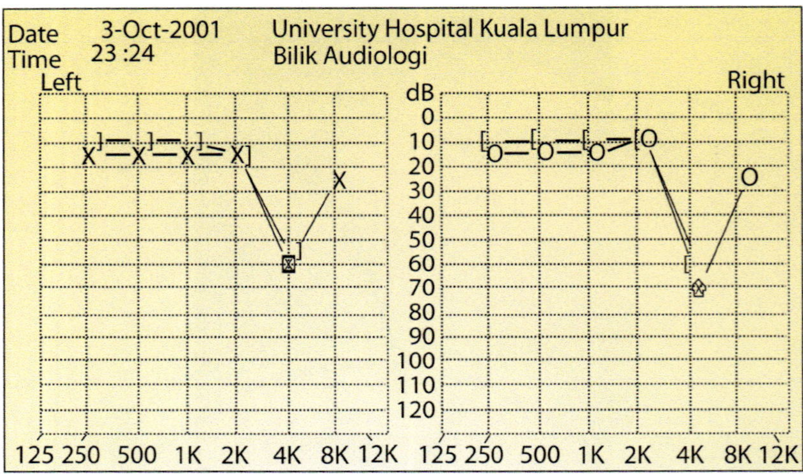

Q. 30. This is the audiogram of a patient who presented with bilateral tinnitus. What is the diagnosis and further management?

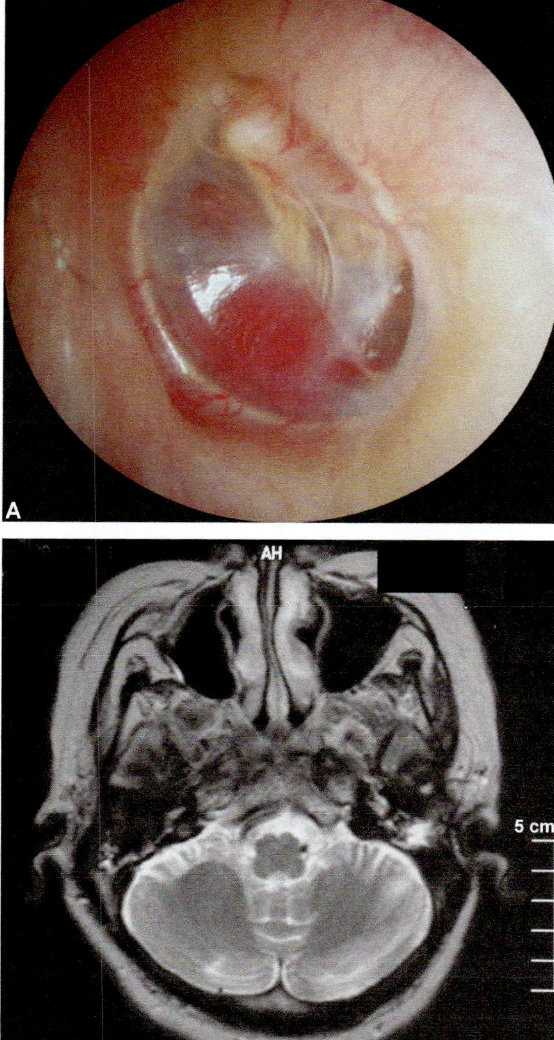

Q. 31. A 69-year-old lady presented with pulsatile tinnitus involving the left ear associated with mild decrease in hearing. Otoscopic examination and subsequent imaging study was ordered.

a. Describe the otoscopic findings.
b. What does the imaging study show?
c. Give the possible diagnoses.
d. Outline the treatment.

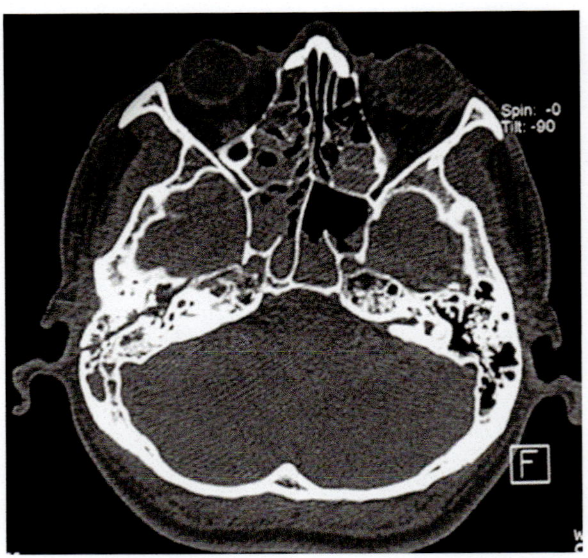

Q. 32. A 37-year-old man was involved in motorcycle accident and sustained head injury needing temporary intensive care. He was referred for ENT evaluation and further assessment.

a. Describe the imaging study findings.
b. What is the diagnosis?
c. List the possible complications from this lesion.
d. How should this patient be managed further?

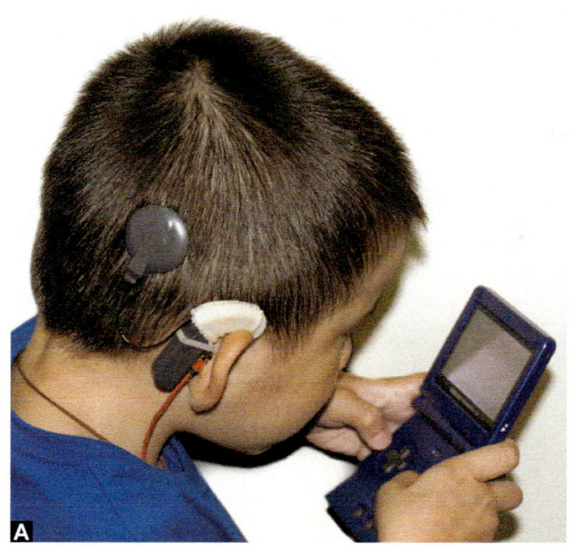

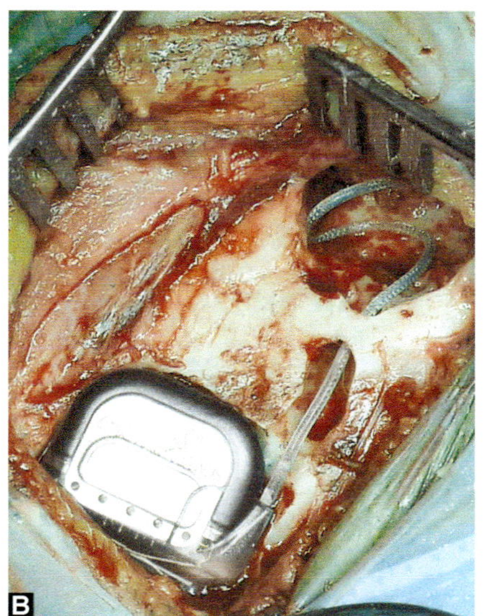

Q. 33. This child had surgery done for profound hearing loss. Related intraoperative images were as shown.

a. What surgery was performed?
b. List its indications.
c. What are the necessary preoperative evaluations needed to be done?
d. How would this child be monitored postoperatively?

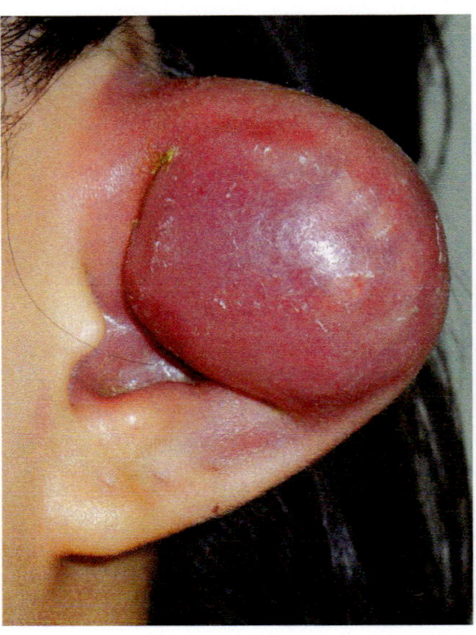

Q. 34. A 17-year-old teenager presented with an increasingly painful left ear swelling of 5 days duration. She admitted to have scratched the pinna due to itchiness, but denied having any recent injury or ear piercing procedure done.

a. Describe the findings.
b. Give the most likely diagnosis.
c. How would this lesion be managed further?
d. List potential complications that can occur.

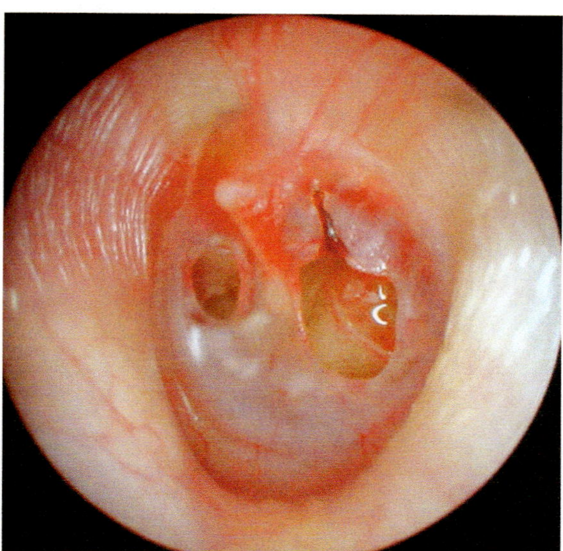

Q. 35. A patient presented to outpatient otolaryngology clinic with complains of painful left ear associated with humming sounds. Further history revealed he had quarreled with a friend and ended with a fight.

a. Describe the otoendoscopic findings.
b. What are the roles of hearing test and audiometry in this instance?
c. How would you tell the patient regarding the prognosis?

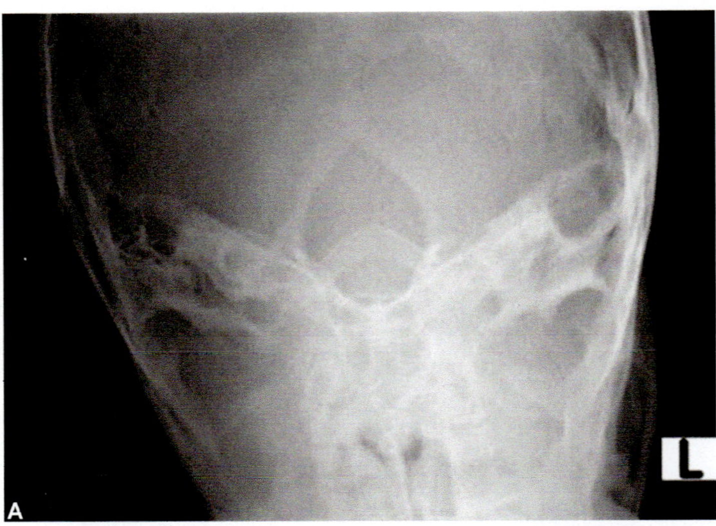

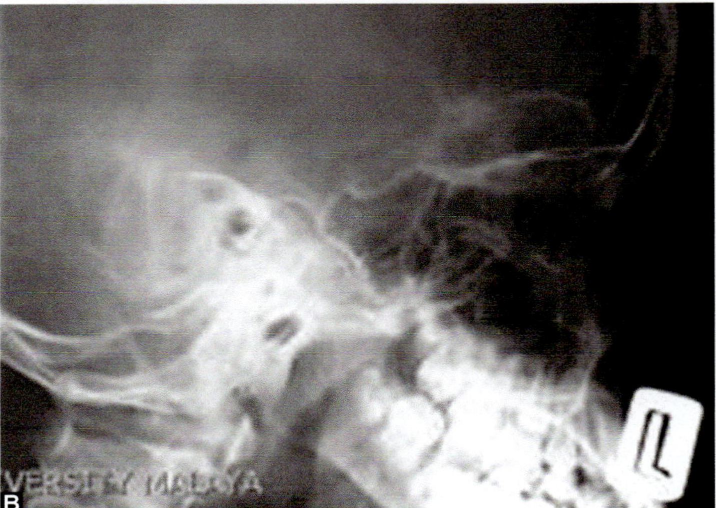

Q. 36. A 14-year-old teenager presented with longstanding history of reduced hearing affecting the left ear. Tuning forks test showed negative Rinne's test on the left with ipsilateral lateralization on Weber's test. X-ray was ordered.

a. Descibe the radiological findings.
b. What is the most likely diagnosis?
c. List its potential complications.
d. How would this patient be managed further?

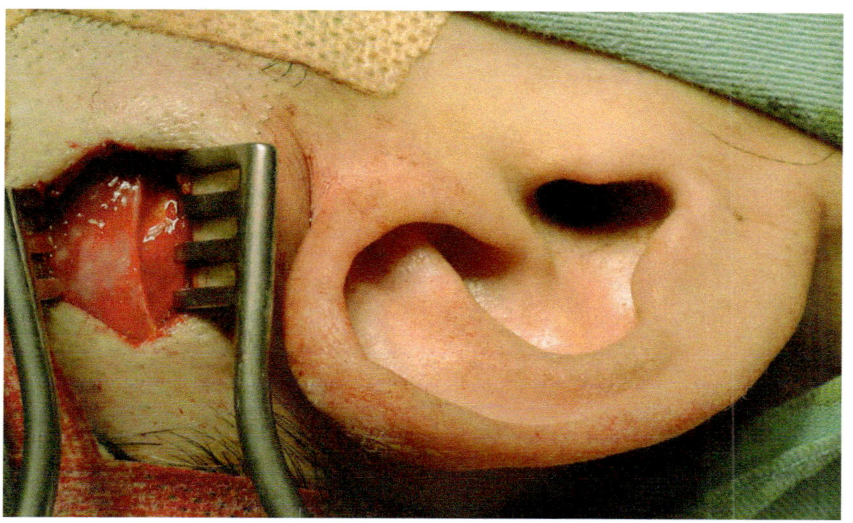

Q. 37. This intraoperative image was taken during a myringoplasty.

a. Describe the step currently being taken.
b. What is its role in myringoplasty?
c. List other materials that can be used for similar purpose.

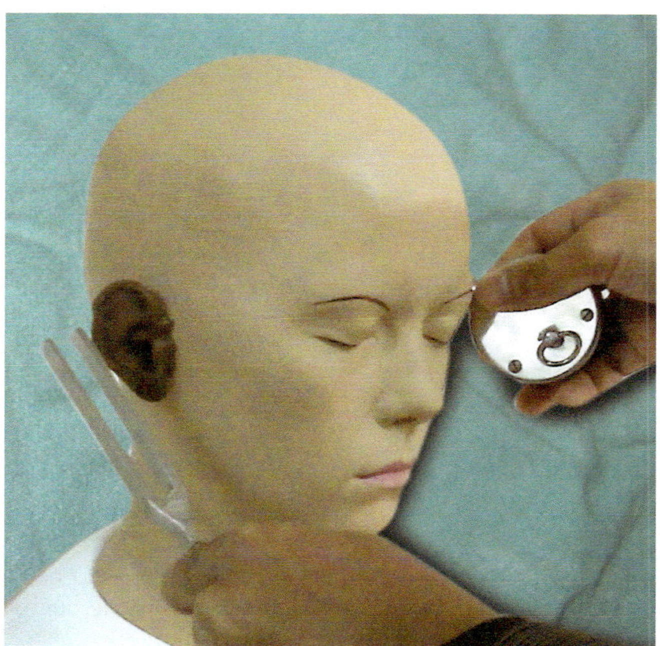

Q. 38. What clinical test is being performed and its significance? Under what circumstances it is necessary?

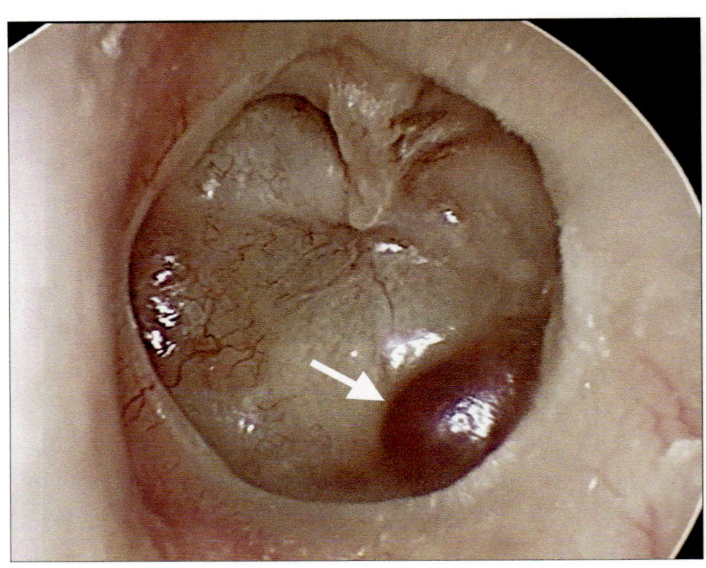

Q. 39. Describe the findings of this otoendoscopic image and give the diagnosis. Identify the structure pointed by the arrow and its significance.

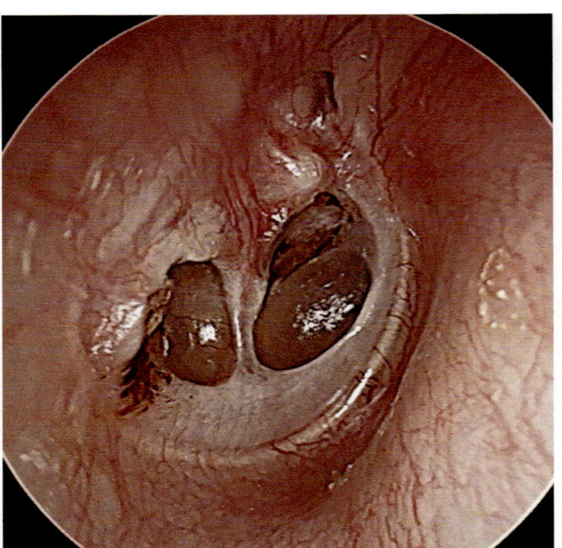

Q. 40. This is an otoendoscopic image of a patient who had previous history of recurrent ear discharge. Presently, he complained of reduced hearing and blocked ear sensation.

a. Describe the findings and give the diagnosis.
b. What is the cause for his hearing loss?
c. How this patient should be managed further?

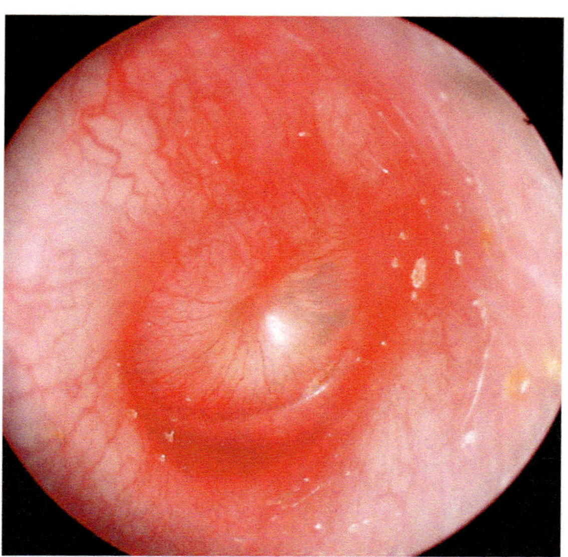

Q. 41. This is the endoscopic finding of the left ear of a child who presented with acute otalgia and blocked ear sensation.

a. Describe the findings and give the diagnosis.

b. List the sequelae of this condition.

c. Outline the treatment.

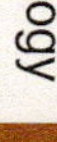

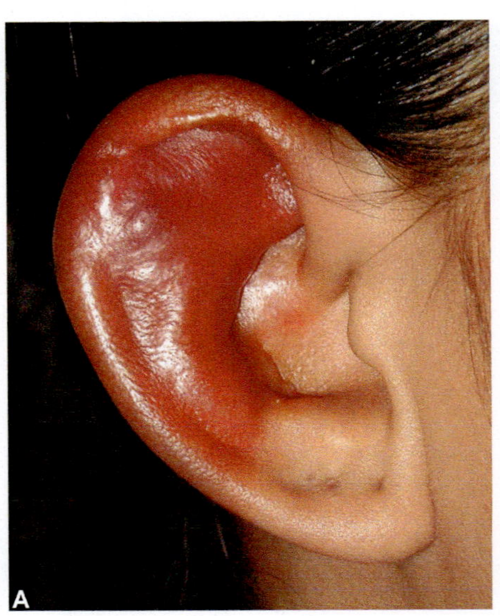

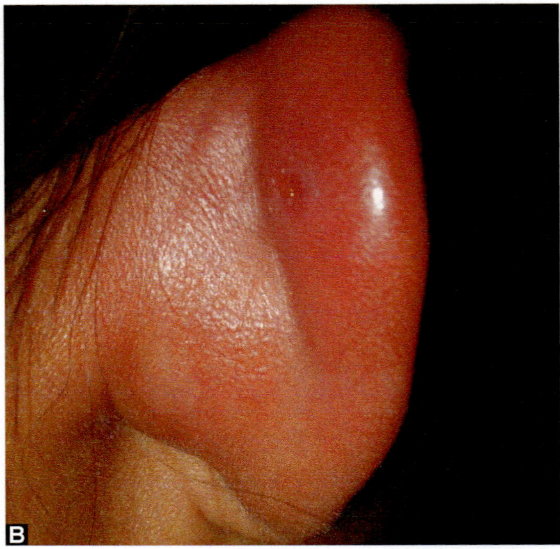

Q. 42. This lady had ear piercing performed by a beautician 3 days prior to consultation. Generally she felt unwell and the pinna feeling hot.

a. Describe the findings and give the diagnosis.
b. List the potential complications that can occur.
c. Outline the treatment.

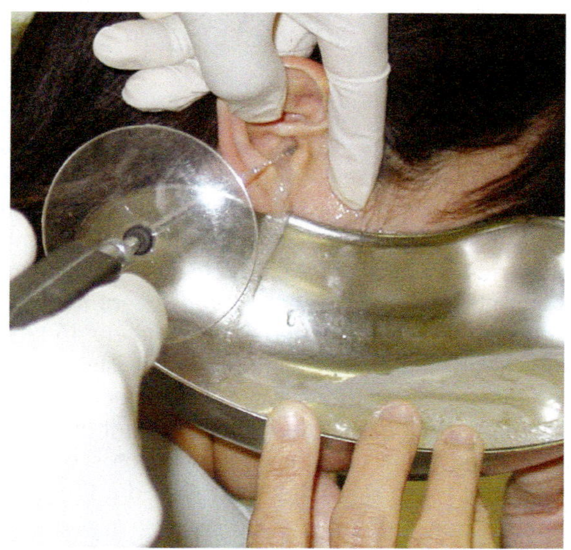

Q. 43. What procedure is being performed? Give its indications. List the potential complications or adverse effects.

Answers

1. This is an endoscopic view of a normal ear canal and left tympanic membrane (TM) (left because the handle of malleus is always directed posteriorly). The ear canal has the characteristic anterior prominence and is free from earwax. This is due to the outward bound epithelial migration that starts from the umbo that radiates out right through the ear canal. Thus, a normal ear is self-cleansing and there is no need to use cotton bud. The TM is pearly translucent in appearance with the handle of malleus positioned approximately 45° to the horizon and the posterior malleolar ligament visible. The cone of light is at the anterior inferior quadrant (around 8 o'clock in the left ear and 4 o'clock in the right ear) as this is the segment of TM that is 90° to the ear canal and thus reflects the light of the otoscope or endoscope. This position of the cone of light is distorted if the TM is abnormal or retracted.

2. a. The normal translucent color of the TM is not present; instead it looks yellowish due to the accumulation of fluid in the middle ear space. The TM is retracted (handle of malleus is more acute than usual 45°) and the Prussak's space is retracted (a potential space just above the lateral process of the malleus). This is consistent with middle ear effusion (MEE) or serous otitis media.

b. The middle ear space is an air-filled cavity that extends posteriorly to the mastoid antrum via the aditus and is connected to the nasopharynx via the Eustachian tube (ET). The ET functions to equalize pressure in the middle ear space and the atmospheric pressure outside. Malfunctions occur most commonly due to mechanical obstruction, which causes a gradual negative pressure development in the middle ear that is eventually filled with fluid.

c. The causes of MEE include ET dysfunction (abnormal ET or muscular movements of ET, e.g. cleft palate, craniofacial abnormalities, mechanical obstruction, e.g. adenoids, tumors [e.g. nasopharyngeal carcinoma (CA), very common cancer in Southeast Asia], allergic rhinitis, and rhinosinusitis, etc.

3. a. This patient has undergone myringotomy and grommet (M&G) insertion.

b. This procedure is indicated for persistent serous otitis media despite conservative management, recurrent acute otitis media, marked ET dysfunction and sometimes for intratympanic gentamicin application in Meniere's disease. This allows the fluid in the middle ear space to be drained, and ventilation regained. As the grommet stays in place for at least a few months, this hopefully will allow the middle ear mucosa to heal and the ET recovers its function and patency before it extrudes.

c. The myringotomy is performed at the anteroinferior quadrant as this is the safest area. Posteroinferior quadrant should be avoided at all cost as the ossicles (long process and lentiform process of incus, stapes), and in some cases dehiscent facial nerve can be injured at this quadrant. Manipulation of the ossicles at this area can also dislocate the stapes footplate and result in a dead ear (total loss of hearing and balance). Severe bleeding can occur in a high jugular bulb, where the jugular bulb occupies the hypotympanum or the lower limit of the middle ear space. A grommet is essentially a tube, thus all complications related to tube applies; it can get blocked, dislodged, and allow fluid from external ear to enter the middle ear space predisposing to frequent middle ear infections. This is commonly seen in children, who swim with their grommets *in situ*.

4. a. The image shows a subtotal central perforation in quiescent stage with the handle and neck of malleus left bare. The long process of incus was absent and the lenticular process of stapes seen surrounded by mucosal adhesions.

b. Rinne's test is expected to be negative and Weber's test lateralized to ipsilateral side indicating conductive hearing loss. As there was ossicular discontinuity on the top of the large perforation, free field voice test and audiometry would reveal severe conductive hearing loss.

c. The options are hearing aid, surgery, or to leave it alone. Surgery needs to be done at several stages including myringoplasty and ossicular prosthesis insertion. The risk of incomplete closure, secondary acquired cholesteatoma, and prosthesis-related complications need to be considered. Care of the ear from contaminants and treatment of intercurrent infections are important along the way.

5. a. This is an abnormal and malformed external ear which is called microtia (micro = small). It is a congenital lesion due to malformation of the first and second branchial arches, which are responsible for external ear formation. It is sometimes associated with absent ear canal, which is called canal atresia as in this case, or a narrow ear canal, e.g. canal stenosis. There is also an accessory skin tag or vestigial auricle.

b. The management of this condition depends on whether the other ear is normal. If the other ear is normal externally and hearing wise, the patient can be advised to wait until he or she is old enough to decide, if they want surgery for cosmetic reason. This is because one functioning ear is enough for the patient to have a normal hearing, speech and education. If the other ear is also abnormal, then the child must have a bone conduction hearing aid or even a bone anchored hearing aid fitted as soon as possible to assist hearing. A computed tomography CT scan is performed at the age of four to rule out any external ear cholesteatoma which will require surgery. The middle ear and mastoid were analyzed for degree of pneumatization and integrity of the ossicular chain, and the normality of inner ear structures determined. A canal reconstruction might be carried out in certain cases with canal atresia. Reconstruction of the pinna can be performed later. Nowadays, there is even bone anchored ear prosthesis that matches the skin color.

6. a. There appears to be a pit or sinus just in front of the helix, which is characteristic of a preauricular sinus. This is also a congenital malformation related to incomplete closure of the branchial arches. Although most commonly found in front of the helix, it can also occur anywhere in the auricle.

b. They are usually asymptomatic. Sometimes, it can become infected and exude purulent discharge. This can also result in an abscess formation with a tender, fluctuant swelling which can be accompanied by fever. The management depends on the presentation. In asymptomatic patients, it can be left alone. In infected cases, antibiotics may be required. Abscess needs drainage and antibiotics, and subsequently requires an excision to completely remove the sinus and its underlying tract in the soft tissue. Inadequate excision of the tract can cause recurrent infection. In rare cases, preauricular sinus is associated with ossicular abnormalities known as Wildervanck syndrome.

7. a. The picture shows a keloid of the pinna. It can occur in anyone, although more commonly in darker skin people. It usually occurs after an injury or any trauma. The fundamental underlying pathology is an exaggerated healing response which causes fibrosis out of the boundaries of the actual injury. These swellings are firm and nontender.

b. Small lesions can be managed by multiple frequent injections of steroids into the swellings while the larger ones will require surgical excision, pressure bandage and subsequent steroid injections (as justified). However, the keloid can still recur despite the best possible management.

8. a. There appears to be a swelling at the external ear canal in the bony segment (the medial aspect of the external ear). This is most likely to be an exostosis. It is due to the bony outgrowth believed to be caused by swimming in cold water. This can be confirmed by palpating the swelling which will be bony hard in consistency. The differential diagnosis includes tumors of the skin appendages, e.g. seboma, etc.

b. In asymptomatic patients, it can be left alone. Surgical management will be required in patients with obstructive symptoms, or in whom where there is a difficulty to clean the ears with resulting earwax cumulation and impaction. The exostosis can be drilled off but there may be a risk of facial nerve palsy.

9. a. Examination revealed left Bell's sign and the pinna appeared erythematous with multiple blisters containing clear fluid.
   b. Ramsay Hunt syndrome or herpes zoster oticus, which is varicella-zoster virus infection involving the geniculate ganglion of facial nerve in the temporal bone.
   c. Laboratory test, e.g. total white count and erythrocyte sedimentation rate can differentiate infective and inflammatory nature of the lesions. Neurological studies has little role and not usually ordered in typical presentation. Pain relief medications are given either orally or by applying local anesthetic. Eye protection is necessary to prevent corneal keratitis; however, this teenager showed positive Bell's sign, which had made the cornea completely concealed. Corticosteroid in tapering doses and acyclovir are the main mode of treatment. The latter has been shown to reduce pain and promote resolution of symptoms if given within 48 hours of symptoms onset.
10. a. The otoscopic view reveals wax almost totally occluding the ear canal.
   b. Usually, the complaint of hearing loss in patients with earwax occurs after swimming or digging the ears. Swimming or entry of water into the ears causes the wax to expand and totally occlude the external ear. This can be uncomfortable with a sense of ear obstruction, which a child will complain of pain and not obstruction. In some patients, they have dizziness and cases of persistent coughs secondary to wax have also been reported. This is due to the vagus nerve (Arnold's nerve) irritation as the nerve supply the innervation to both (tympanic membrane) and the larynx.
   c. In a child with impacted wax, removal either by syringing or direct vision (under microscope) can be difficult due to the lack of cooperation as the procedure can be painful. It is better to instill wax softener, e.g. cerumol for few days to soften and dissolve the wax before the procedure is undertaken. Syringing should not be performed if the TM is suspected to be perforated.
11. a. There is a yellow round object at the opening of the ear canal most likely a foreign body. Foreign body of the ear can be divided into organic and non-organic. Organic foreign body can lead to infection and need to be removed quickly. Insects, if alive can be extremely painful and need to be killed with the use of any liquid. Non-organic foreign body can be asymptomatic and left unnoticed for some time.
   b. The management of ear foreign body is by removal. A round object would require a probe or a curved hook to be inserted behind it, while the flat foreign bodies can be removed with the forceps. Syringing can be used although if not used in the right method can cause the foreign body to be pushed further inside. Some cases of tightly impacted foreign body may require removal under general anesthesia. Injuries to the TM or ossicles have been

reported in overzealous or unskillful attempt at the removal of impacted foreign bodies.

12. This is a typical otoscopic view of otomycosis or fungal infection of the ear. The black spores seen in the picture indicate *Aspergillus niger*, while the white plague is often candidiasis. Together they form a 'wet newspaper' appearance. Otomycosis is predominantly seen in humid tropical countries like Malaysia. Frequent, recurrent otomycosis should be investigated for the possibility of diabetes mellitus. The presentation can vary from itchiness and pain to a sensation of blockage. Management involves a thorough cleaning of the ear, typically under the microscope with a meticulous attention to the inferior recess area. Antifungal ear drops, ointment, or powder can then be used topically for at least 6 weeks.

13. This otoscopic picture reveals a central perforation (around 30%) with purulent discharge noted around 9 o'clock and the inferior recess area. Thus, this indicates an active stage of chronic suppurative otitis media (CSOM). The term tubotympanic (TT) indicates that the perforation is safe that it does not have cholesteatoma and the possible complications that can arise from it. However, TT is often not used and other term that can be used to describe this condition includes CSOM (safe), CSOM mucosal disease or just CSOM without cholesteatoma. In the presence of active discharge, a thorough ear toilet is performed followed by topical antibiotic drops or even oral antibiotic if justified. The patient will be advised to keep his ear dry and subsequently, once it remains dry for a period of at least 2–3 months, myringoplasty can be safely performed. Preoperative audiogram is taken for record keeping. If the ear continues to discharge despite antibiotics (after culture and sensitivity), then cortical mastoidectomy needs to be considered. This is to clear the infected mastoid air cells which would have served as a reservoir for the persistent infection. (Note: Small perforation can close by itself overtime provided the ear is dry and devoid of infection thus not always need a repair).

14. a. There is an attic (area above the anterior and posterior malleolar ligament or pars flaccida and scutum) pocket with white flaky debris characteristic of cholesteatoma. The pars tensa appears normal.

b. The discharge in these patients tends to be persistent, scanty, and foul-smelling as compared to intermittent, copious, mucopurulent, odorless discharge of CSOM (TT). Thus, the diagnosis is CSOM [atticoantral (AA)]. Atticoantral indicates that the perforation is unsafe; that it does have cholesteatoma and the possible complications that can arise from it. However, AA is often not used and other terms that can be used to describe this condition include CSOM (unsafe), CSOM epithelial disease or just CSOM with cholesteatoma.

c. The management of this condition is essential to prevent the possible complications if it is allowed to expand; namely brain abscess, labyrinthitis, facial palsy, subperiosteal abscess and sigmoid sinus thrombosis. In a small cavity and a medically unfit patient, regular cleaning will be adequate if all the boundaries of the sac or cavity can be visualized and easily assessed with the help of a microscope. If this is not possible, mastoid exploration and exteriorization of cholesteatoma should be carried out. This can be divided into an atticotomy, modified radical mastoidectomy (MRM) or combined approach mastoidectomy depending on the severity and intraoperative findings.

15. a. This is a left (the handle of malleus always points backward giving a clue to if the ear is right or left) otoendoscopic view that reveals a dark fluid collection in the middle ear space, probably blood. The posterior malleolar ligament is also prominent with retraction of the attic (Prussak's space) observed indicating the possibility of a negative middle ear pressure. There appears to be a healed perforation at around 7 o'clock (anteroinferior aspect) suggesting this patient might have had a grommet inserted before.

b. This finding is typically seen in hemotympanum. In this condition, there is a collection of blood in the middle ear space usually resulting from trauma. In some cases, it occurs secondary to severe barotrauma when sudden changes of pressure occur while flying or scuba diving in the presence of a nonfunctioning ET. This causes an acute marked negative middle ear pressure with collection of fluid or even blood in severe cases. Similar appearance can also be found in cholesterol granuloma with MEE.

c. Hemotympanum is usually self-resolving and no surgical intervention is necessary. Decongestants may be prescribed and patient is advised to perform Valsalva maneuver if possible. Antibiotic is not necessary. In a patient, without history of trauma, middle ear fluid obtained upon myringotomy can be sent for pathological examination if cholesterol granuloma is suspected and, thereafter, the patient treated accordingly.

16. a. This picture reveals a post MRM cavity where mastoid, attic and the external ear were operated and joined together to form a single chamber. It is usually performed to exteriorize the cholesteatoma to render the 'unsafe' ear into 'safe ear'. The middle ear cavity is usually closed off by laying the TM over the medial aspect of middle ear space since the scutum has been removed. This is important as an open middle ear cavity with its respiratory mucosa (goblets cells and other mucous secreting glands) will cause a discharging mastoid cavity. In MRM, the facial ridge is lowered sufficiently to prevent 'sump' effect in the mastoid bowl.

b. Complications of this surgery include injury to the dura [with or without cerebrospinal fluid (CSF) leak], labyrinth, facial nerve and sigmoid sinus. There can also be a profound hearing loss that is believed due to the drills used during the surgery.

c. Other procedures include atticotomy and combined approach tympanoplasty. In atticotomy, disease that is limited to the attic is removed by removing the scutum and exteriorizing the attic pocket. This can be reconstructed with a cartilage grafting the same sitting if the surgeon is confident that all the cholesteatoma has been removed or perform later in the second sitting. Combined approach tympanoplasty or canal wall up procedure is usually performed in children, with well-pneumatized mastoid and in patients, who complaint and understand that this is a two-stage procedure. This procedure prevents a mastoid cavity and its complications (discharging ear, regular ear toileting for life, vertigo and imbalance in cold winds) and retains a normal external ear canal. It can be technically more challenging as a posterior tympanotomy (boundary: facial nerve, chorda tympani and buttress) is performed together with the elevation of a tympanomeatal flap to remove the disease. As recurrence rate is high, a second look is vital.

17. The right otoscopic view reveals an intact (tympanic membrane) with a bulging mass behind it between 9 o'clock and 12 o'clock position. The mass appears to be white in color and the presence of blood vessels running over the mass continuous with the ear canal confirms the presence of an intact TM. This appears to be a congenital cholesteatoma, which refers to the persistence of embryonic epithelial cell crest in the middle ear cleft. Congenital cholesteatoma can also occur in petrous apex, cerebellopontine (CP) angle and mastoid. Since the TM is intact, they do not present with the typical scanty, purulent, persistent foul-smelling discharge that is the characteristic of CSOM (AA). Thus, their main presenting symptom is usually hearing loss or facial nerve palsy depending on the size and location of the cholesteatoma. Management consists of a pure tone audiogram (PTA) to assess and document the extent of hearing loss and a high resolution computed tomographic (HRCT) scan that will be able to assess the location, extent and other anatomical configurations that are important in planning the gold standard of treatment: surgical Excision.

18. a. This otoendoscopy view of the left ear reveals an adhesive otitis media. It usually occurs as a consequence of chronic ET dysfunction that leads to chronic persistent negative middle ear pressure. Eventually, the TM will be sucked in and draped or even adherent to the medial aspect of the middle ear. The following structures can be identified:

- Handle of malleus
- Lateral process of malleus
- Umbo
- Promontory
- Round window niche

- Long process of incus
- Head of stapes
- Stapedius tendon.

b. The hearing loss is minimal as the TM is draped and adherent to the stapes forming a natural type III tympanoplasty (natural myringostapediopexy). The presence of an intact TM prevents a discharging ear.

c. Management of this condition needs to address two main factors. The ET and the nasopharynx should be examined to rule out any pathology and managed accordingly. As for the sensation of fullness, M&G can be attempted if there is enough room to insert one. With regards to the hearing loss, if it is significant and impairing the quality of life of the patient, a hearing aid would probably be the best solution. Surgical exploration and attempts to reventilate the middle ear by elevating the TM is often unsuccessful with the reformation of adhesions.

19. The otoendoscopy reveals an opaque TM with an anteroinferior area atrophic (thinner) segment (estimated 20%), which indicates a healed perforation. The location of the atrophic segment suggests possibility of a previous grommet insertion site or probably a central perforation complicating CSOM. The opaque TM indicates thickening and scarring, and thus suggests frequent or longstanding middle ear infection previously. Although the TM is intact, the atrophic segment would not be able to vibrate as good as a normal TM and the energy transmitted to the ossicles would be reduced. Audiogram will show the severity of hearing loss. The management would be to advise the use of hearing aid if the hearing loss is significant. There is no role of surgery in this condition.

20. a. This is an endoscopic view of the left ear, where there appears to be a white structure beneath the TM that appears to be thicker than an abnormal TM. The attic region appears to be retracted and could possibly have undergone surgery.

b. Based on the appearance, there are two possibilities. The white structure could be the cartilage that was used (or even two pieces of cartilage) that is usually used to reconstruct the attic after an atticotomy, or the other possibility is that of incus interposition in an ossiculoplasty or tympanoplasty.

21. a. The endoscopic view reveals a red, fleshy mass with surrounding mucopus in the external ear canal. This appears to be an aural polyp. It can occur due to infection, cholesteatoma, malignant otitis externa, or even malignancy.

b. In this patient, ear swab was taken for culture and sensitivity, and thereafter, a thorough aural toilet and examination under microscope was performed. It is important to probe all around the polyp to see where the stalk or where the polyp is coming from. If it is arising from middle ear, the probe will be able to go all around the polyp. A trial of antibiotic can be given and subsequently polypectomy carried out using a snare. If it is arising from the posterosuperior aspect, then there is a strong possibility of cholesteatoma and a mastoid exploration after CT scan would be required. Biopsy of the polyp is taken to rule out any malignancy.

22. a. There appears to be a red, granular mass in the introitus of the left ear canal. Considering the age of the patient (white hair!) and the presenting symptom of bleeding, a malignancy, e.g. CA of the ear would be the provisional diagnosis. Differential diagnosis would include ear polypor granulation. The presence of facial nerve palsy would usually support the diagnosis of CA ear.

b. Management would consist of a thorough ear toilet and examination under microscope if possible, biopsy and a high definition CT scan. If biopsy confirms malignancy, CT scan should be assessed to look for the involvement of mastoid, middle and inner ear, and the extension beyond the temporal bone including neck metastasis, parotid gland and temporomandibular joint. Surgical management would depend on the extent of local involvement ranging from a sleeve resection for an ear canal CA, a lateral temporal bone resection if the inner ear is not involved (removal of all bone and tissue lateral to facial nerve and closure of ear canal in a blind sac fashion), a subtotal or total temporal bone resection if inner ear is involved, and a combined neck dissection with parotidectomy if these are involved. Radiotherapy is given postoperatively. The prognosis is quite poor for extensive lesions.

23. a. This is an axial CT scan of the skull base and temporal bone (bony window).

b. (1) Mastoid air cells (well-pneumatized), (2) Jugular bulb, (3) Pneumatization of zygoma, (4) Ossicles, (5) Cochlea, (6) Sphenoid sinuses, (7) Internal carotid artery [horizontal (right) and vertical (left) portion in petrous apex], (8) Sigmoid sinus and (9) External auditory canal.

24. a. This is a coronal view of magnetic resonance imaging (MRI) scan most probably with gadolinium. It reveals a lesion at the CP angle most likely due to a vestibular schwannoma (VS) [also commonly known as acoustic neuroma].

b. The differential diagnoses of CP angle mass include meningioma, aneurysm, cholesteatoma and cholesterol granuloma. However, the presence of an extension of the tumor into the internal auditory meatus (IAM) is almost pathognomonic for VS (as seen in this image). Meningiomas are usually more broad based, does not extend into the IAM and frequently has a dural tail.

c. The clinical presentation of a VS ranges from purely otological symptoms in early stage to neurological in more advanced stage. In early cases, where the tumor is localized in the IAM (usually < 2 cm), patients present with asymmetrical hearing loss or occasionally sudden hearing loss. Occasionally, tinnitus and imbalance can be the presenting symptoms. In larger lesion (> 2 cm), cranial nerve symptoms (fifth, seventh and ninth, tenth) can be present. The earliest being loss of corneal reflex and paresthesia of the cheek (trigeminal nerve). Cerebellar compression causes imbalance and brainstem compression can be eventually fatal. Large lesions can cause hydrocephalus. They rarely present with facial nerve palsy.

d. Management takes into account multiple factors including age, hearing level, general medical condition and the patient's preference of treatment. This ranges from observation with yearly MRI for small lesion (1.5 cm) (Note: acoustic neuroma is a slow growing tumor), radiosurgery for lesions below 2–2.5 cm in elderly patients, and surgical removal in patients with large tumors that indents the brainstem and cerebellum.

25. This appears to be an endoscopic view of the right TM. The pars flaccida (attic) is retracted, specifically at the area of Prussak's space (above the lateral process of the handle of malleus, scutum and the neck of malleus). There is an evidence of previous M&G insertion with the presence of a healed perforation (TM thinner than normal) at around 4 o'clock. The yellowish discoloration over the healed perforation can be due to adhesion to the promontory or the presence of serous otitis media (glue ear). This is typically seen in longstanding ET obstruction commonly from childhood itself. These patients usually present with sensation of ear fullness and blockage, inability to equalize the ears, and in some cases hearing loss.

26. Brainstem evoked response audiometry (BERA). It is an objective audiological testing, wherein sound stimulus generates electrical responses in the cochlea (inner ear) and in the brainstem. This response travels along the auditory pathway, resulting in waveforms, identifiable to the site of origin by the amplitude and latency. The advantages of BERA include noninvasive, reliability on repetitive testing, and not affected by sedatives or drugs. Thus, it is most useful in newborn and neonates. In adult, it is mostly ordered for acoustic neuroma, to differentiate cochlear and retrocochlear lesion, and in malingering patients.

27. a. Conductive hearing loss in the presence of normal TM suggests a middle ear pathology. These may range from tympanosclerosis, ossicular discontinuity, adhesion, or even ossicular fusion. This patient is very likely to have otosclerosis, a condition whereby there is a new bone formation at or about the stapes footplate thus impeding the transmission of sound to the oval window. The lesion is more commonly found in females and hormonal changes during pregnancy would have accelerated the disease process.

b. Figure A shows a complete stapes structure, i.e. the footplate, anterior and posterior crus, and its head. Figure B shows a whitish material encircling and anchored at the lower part of the long process of incus.

c. These figures gave a clue to stapedectomy with tympanoplasty performed. Ossicular reconstruction can be done with various commercialized materials, e.g. titanium piston, or synthetic material such as plastipore (likely in this case since it is white in color). This would restore the sound transmission to the round window enabling closure of air-bone gap.

28. a. Figure A showed mastoid and postauricular skin bruise, the typical Battle's sign while Figure B showed a bluish spherical rim in the middle ear (an indicator of resolving hemotympanum) and purplish bruise along and around the handle of malleus with no obvious clue of ear canal injury. These signs are highly suggestive of skull base fractures involving the squamous temporal bone (usually transverse fracture if TM is intact). In contrast, the presence of these findings in infant and young children would be suspicious of nonaccidental injury or child abuse.

b. Cranial nerves examination in particular, the facial and auditory nerves, to document paralysis and hearing loss, respectively. Presence of conductive hearing loss without immediate facial palsy, sensorineural hearing loss (SNHL), or vestibular symptoms are in favor of longitudinal fractures rather than transverse fractures of the temporal bone.

c. In this patient, there is no facial palsy or nystagmus noted and the hearing loss is mild and conductive in nature, thus a conservative management is chosen.

29. This is typical of a subperiosteal abscess that is seen as a complication of acute mastoiditis. This can be an emergency condition. This child needs admission, intravenous antibiotics, CT scan to rule out intracranial complication (upto 30% of the children can have asymptomatic intracranial complication) with the definitive treatment of surgical exploration of the mastoid. The postauricular incision should be higher in children due to the incomplete elongation of the mastoid tip as the facial nerve can be injured in a normally placed postauricular incision.

30. This is a PTA of a patient performed in October 2001. It reveals a dip at 4 kHz of upto 60–70 decibel (dB) with normal hearing threshold in all other frequencies. This is typically seen in noise-induced hearing loss. The dip at 4 kHz is believed to be due to the fact that the promontory (corresponds to 4 kHz) is the most sensitive part of the cochlea, therefore, vulnerable to noise insults. It initially presents as a temporary threshold shift (in early stage) that recovers to normal hearing threshold. Permanent damage leads to a similar audiogram as above. This is usually due to the exposure of noise above 90 dB, 8 hours a day, 5 days a week. If this patient is working in a noisy environment, it is vital that he is referred to occupational health authorities and provided with appropriate ear protection while working.

31. a. Otoscopic examination reveals a reddish mass in the inferior part of the left middle ear behind the intact TM. This appears to be arising from the floor of the middle ear, extending to the umbo.

b. This MRI shows a hyperintense or hypervascular mass at the left middle ear space. It seems to be localized in this area without any extension into mastoid air cells.

c. The possible diagnosis includes glomus tympanicum, glomus jugulare and possibly high jugular bulb.

d. The main treatment is excision of the lesion. She needs a preoperative angiogram and embolization to reduce the risk of bleeding from the lesion intraoperatively. The other option is conservative, especially if the lesion is not growing and the patient is not fit for surgery.

32. a. This HRCT scan shows a longitudinal fracture of right temporal bone from ear canal toward the petrous apex, traversing the middle ear space with soft tissue density at the right mastoid cavity, most likely blood accumulation after temporal bone fracture.

b. The diagnosis is a longitudinal fracture of right temporal bone with hematoma.

c. The possible complications from this lesion include conductive hearing loss, facial nerve palsy, vertigo and CSF leak.

d. The management is usually conservative and depends on the complications of the fracture. Delayed onset of facial nerve paralysis is treated conservatively, while immediate onset of total facial paralysis may require surgery in the form of decompression, reanastomosis of cut ends or cable graft. Hearing test is always needed during follow-up to assess any hearing loss. Neurotological examination and assessment is important as labyrinth concussion may occur.

33. a. This child has had right cochlear implant performed.

b. The indications of cochlear implants include severe to profound bilateral SNHL (unaided threshold >90 dB) with little or no benefit from 3 months to 4 months trial of hearing aid. This may be performed for congenital hearing loss in children ideally before the age of four or in postlingual deafness in adults or older children. Children with congenital hearing loss detected after the age of four may not have good results.

c. The necessary preoperative evaluations include trial of hearing aid for 3–6 months, no medical contraindication to undergo surgery, good family support, preoperative HRCT to assess the anatomy of the inner ear, otoscopic examination to rule out any middle ear infection and assessment by audiologist and speech therapist.

d. The child needs to be followed up with the experienced audiologist and speech therapist for cochlear implant rehabilitation. This is probably the most crucial part of the program.

34. a. There appears to be a red and angry looking swelling of superior part of the left pinna.

b. This is most likely a left pinna abscess.

c. The patient needs to be admitted for hydration, intravenous antibiotics and later incision and drainage with anesthesia. Corrugated drain needs to be inserted to drain the pus for the next few days. Later, she needs to be followed up with regular daily dressing till the wound is clean and healed. She would require oral antibiotics upon discharge for the perichondritis.

d. The potential complications that can occur includes septicemia, perichondritis and cauliflower ear.

35. a. This otoendoscopic examination reveals two central perforations of left TM, one at anterior quadrant and the other at posterior quadrant with ragged perforation edges and there is blood clot noted at the superior edge of the posterior perforation. The remaining TM appears hyperemic.

b. Hearing test and audiometry are vital to assess the extent of the hearing loss mainly for medical legal documentation as well as comparison during follow-up.

c. The chances of traumatic TM to recover spontaneously are high as long as there is no superimposed infection. However, the hearing and balance will have to be assessed as well as the inner ear function can be compromised in trauma.

36. a. There appears an area of periantral sclerosis, which is typically seen in cholesteatoma.

b. This should be diagnosed as cholesteatoma, until a microscopic examination reveals otherwise.

c. Cholesteatoma can erode bone and cause intracranial (meningitis, intracranial abscesses) and extracranial (facial nerve palsy, sigmoid sinus thrombosis, labyrinthitis and subperiosteal abscesses) complications.

d. This child will require surgical exploration of the attic and mastoid cavity; most likely a MRM.

37. a. The step shown in this image is harvesting of the temporalis fascia graft for myringoplasty.

b. The role of a graft in myringoplasty is as a scaffold for the epithelium of the perforation edges to epithelialize and close the perforation.

c. Other materials that can be used for similar purpose include perichondrium, cartilage, periosteum and fat tissue.

38. The clinical test that is being performed is masking Rinne tuning fork test. The significance of this test is to mask the non-tested ear with Barany's noise box to decrease the crossover effect from the normal non-tested ear. This test is necessary in severe unilateral SNHL (the right ear in this instance).

39. This is an otoendoscopic image of the left eardrum which shows Grade IV pars tensa retraction with the eardrum adhered to medial wall of the middle ear cavity. The pointed bluish structure is most likely a high jugular bulb which occasionally be seen as an anomaly in this region.

40. a. The otoendoscopic image shows two atrophic central TM retraction. There appears to be straw-colored MEE. This is most likely healed doubled perforations from previous CSOM. Absence of scar made history of previous myringoplasty unlikely.

b. This patient most likely has right conductive hearing loss due to persistent glue ear.

c. Structural and functional cause that gives rise to ET dysfunction need to be ruled out and treated accordingly. Grommet insertion is an alternative measure but the risk of nonclosure should be borne in mind in this paper-thin atrophic healed perforation.

41. a. The otoendoscopic finding is bulging, and hyperemia right TM with loss of cone of light. This is presuppurative stage of acute suppurative otitis media.

b. Sequelae of this condition are TM perforation, nonsuppurative MEE, adhesion, tympanosclerosis, erosion of ossicular chain, and hearing loss (conductive and SNHL).

c. The principles of further management are:

- Antibacterial therapy
- Decongestant nasal drops
- Analgesics and antipyretics
- Myringotomy to be performed when:
  - The eardrum is bulging and there is severe acute pain
  - Incomplete resolution despite antibiotics with the eardrum remains full with persistent conductive hearing loss
  - Persistent effusion beyond 12 weeks.

42. a. These photos show red, swollen right pinna. This is acute right pinna perichondritis.

b. The potential complications that can occur are pinna abscess, sepsis and cauliflower ear.

c. The treatment consists of parenteral antibiotics, analgesic and antipyretics. If abscess develops, incision and drainage needs to be performed.

43. The procedure that is being performed is ear syringing.

The indications of ear syringing are impacted earwax and removal of non-organic foreign body in the ear.

The potential complications include TM perforation, dislocation of ossicular chain, conductive hearing loss, SNHL, acute dizziness, and facial nerve palsy.

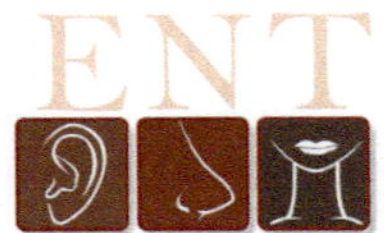

2 RHINOLOGY

Questions

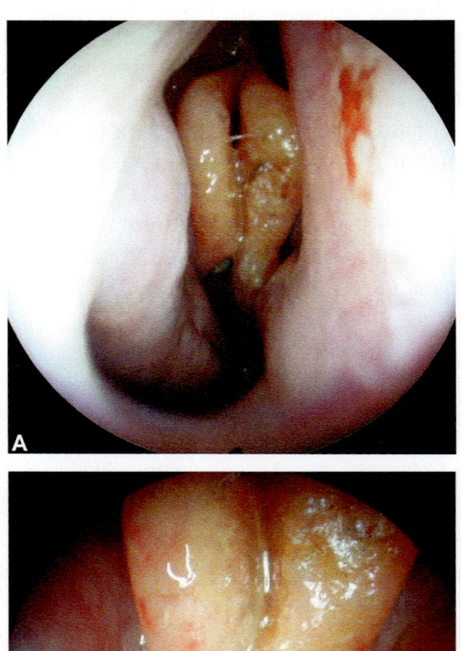

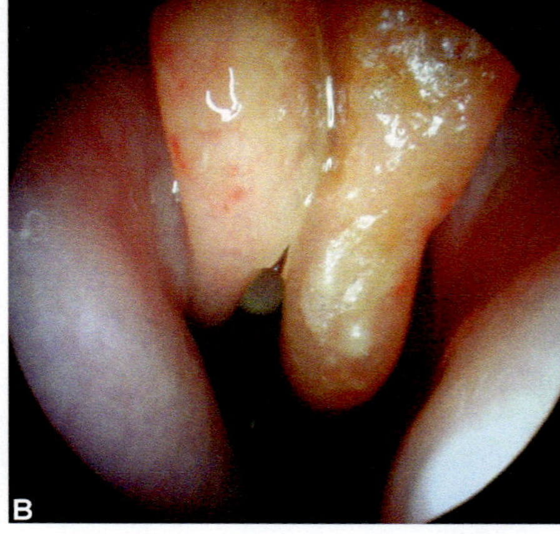

Q. 44. These are endoscopic images of the right nasal cavity.

a. What does it show?
b. What is the clinical implication?
c. How would this patient be managed subsequently?

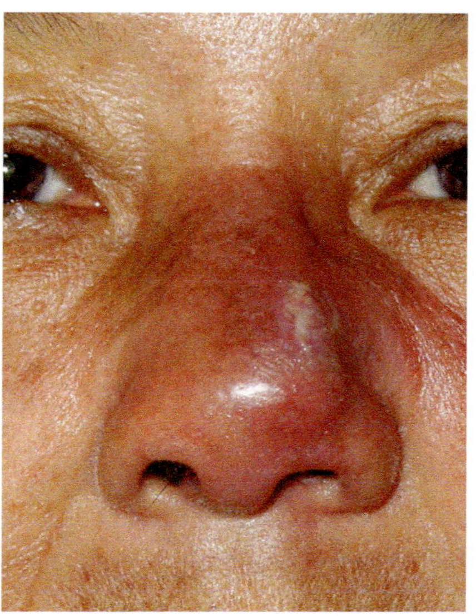

Q. 45. This patient presented with painful, tender nose.

a. What is the diagnosis?
b. What are the possible complications?
c. Outline this patient's management.

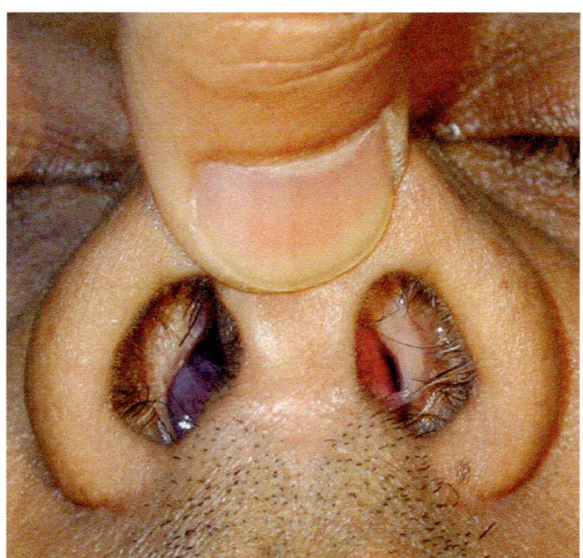

Q. 46. This patient presented with a longstanding history of nasal obstruction bilaterally.

a. What does this examination reveal?
b. How should this patient be managed further?

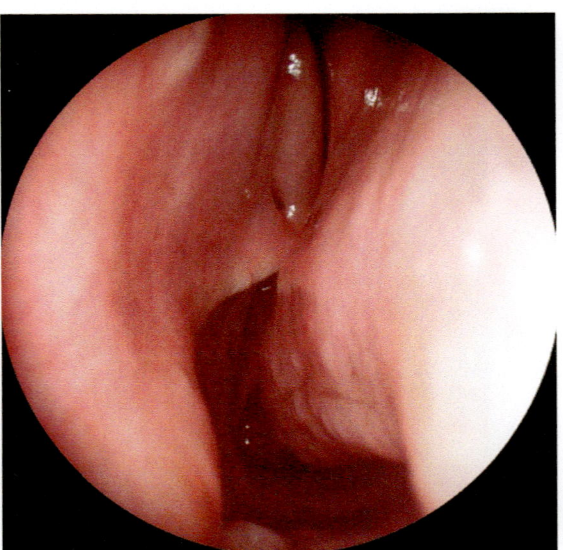

Q. 47. This is a view obtained during an endoscopic nasal examination of the left nasal cavity.

a. What is the abnormality?
b. What are the possible clinical implications?
c. How would this lesion be managed?

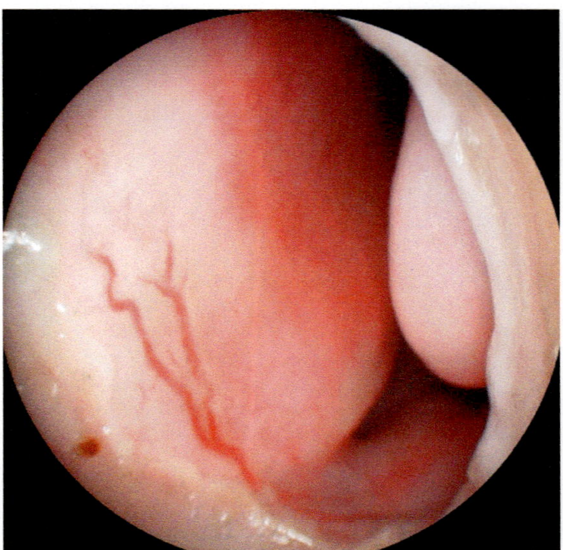

Q. 48. This patient presented with recurrent bleeding from the left nostril.

a. What is the diagnosis?
b. How would this patient be managed further?

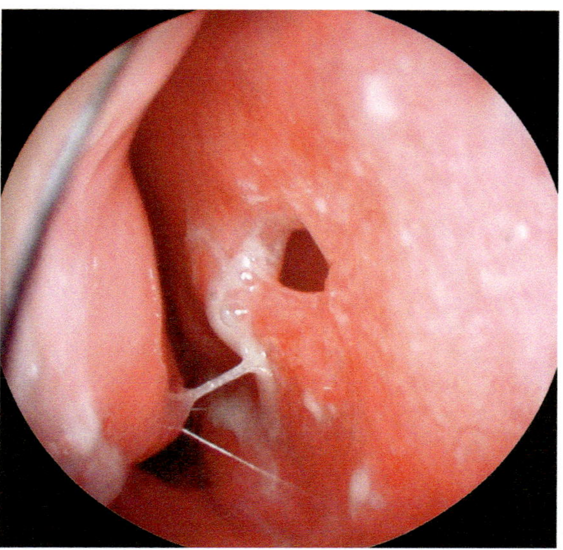

Q. 49. This patient was seen in the clinic with nasal symptoms.

a. What are the diagnoses and its possible etiologies?
b. What are the clinical manifestations?
c. How would this condition be managed further?

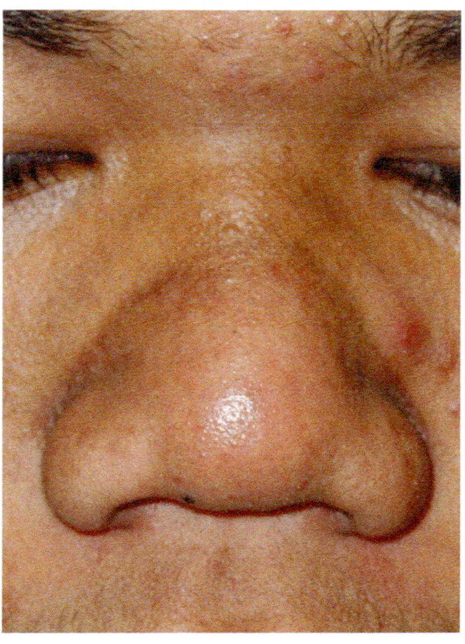

Q. 50. The above patient was seen in an allergy clinic.

a. What is the sign demonstrated?
b. What is the cause?

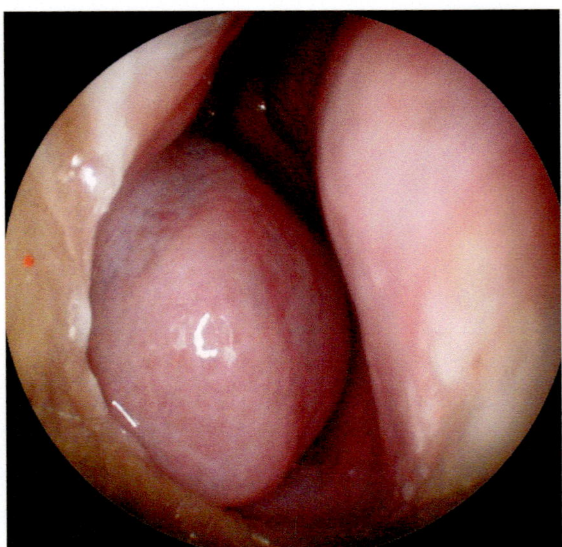

Q. 51. This is the nasal endoscopic view of a patient who presented with nasal obstruction.

a. What does this image show?
b. What are the possible etiologies?
c. What further treatment would be necessary?

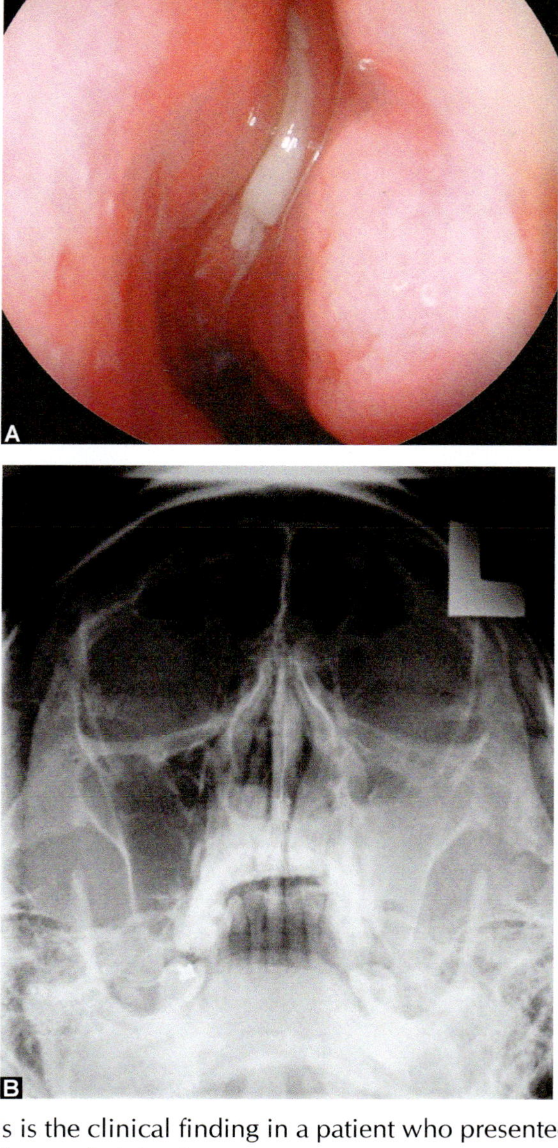

Q. 52. This is the clinical finding in a patient who presented with fever and acute facial pain.

a. What is the diagnosis?

b. Outline the subsequent treatment.

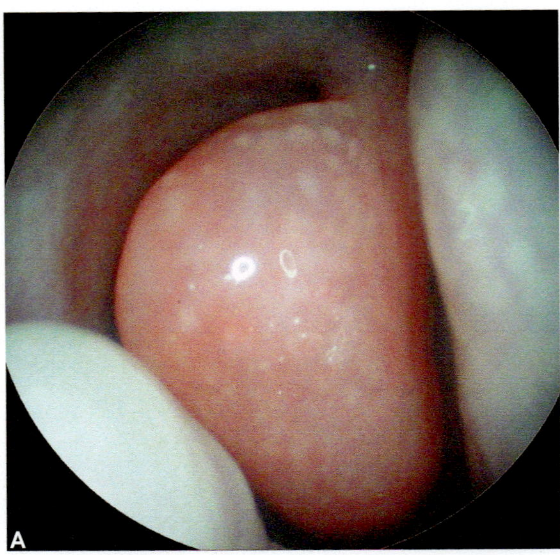

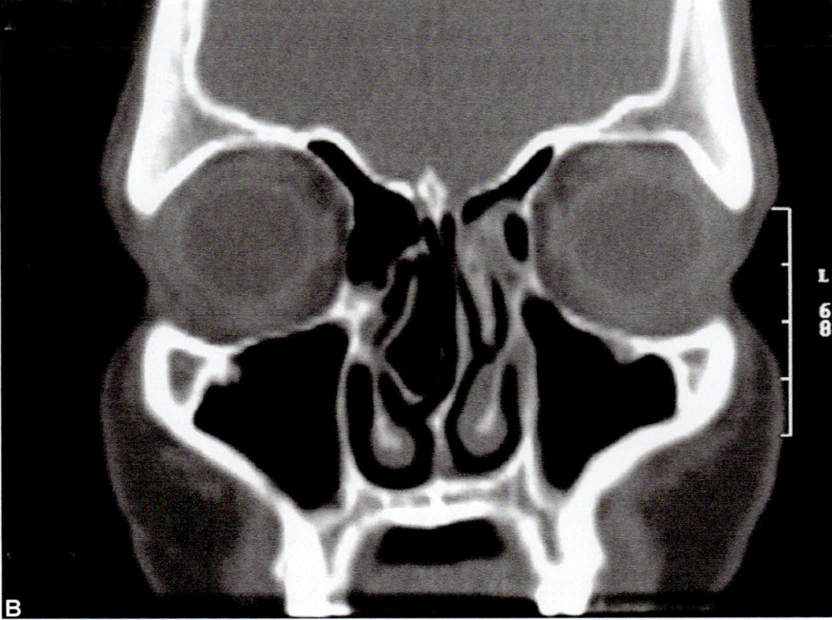

Q. 53. The above patient presented with recurrent acute sinusitis. Endoscopic finding and computed tomography scan of the paranasal sinuses are enclosed.

a. What is the diagnosis?

b. Outline the management of this patient.

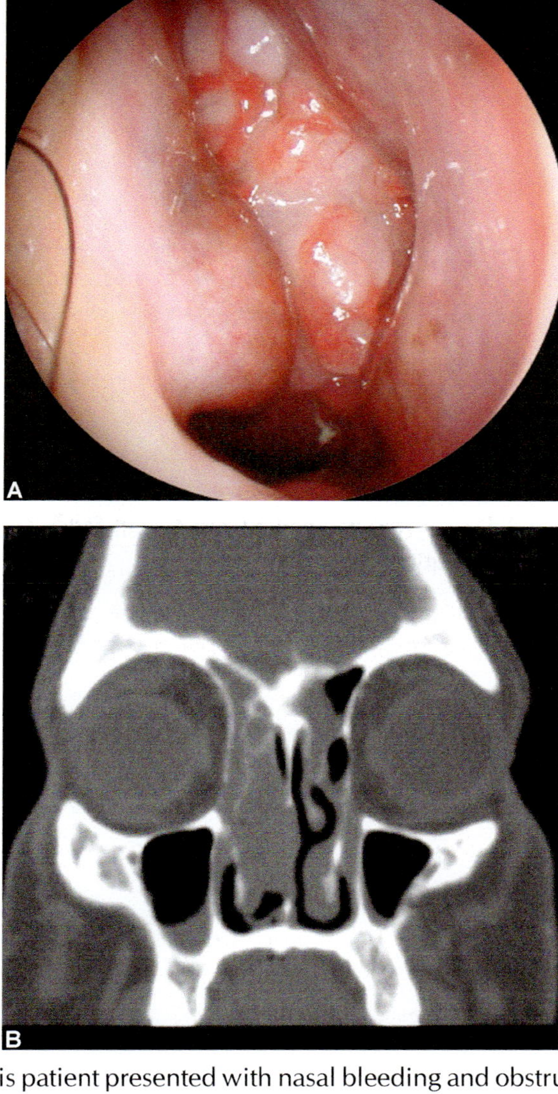

Q. 54. This patient presented with nasal bleeding and obstruction. What is the diagnosis and its management?

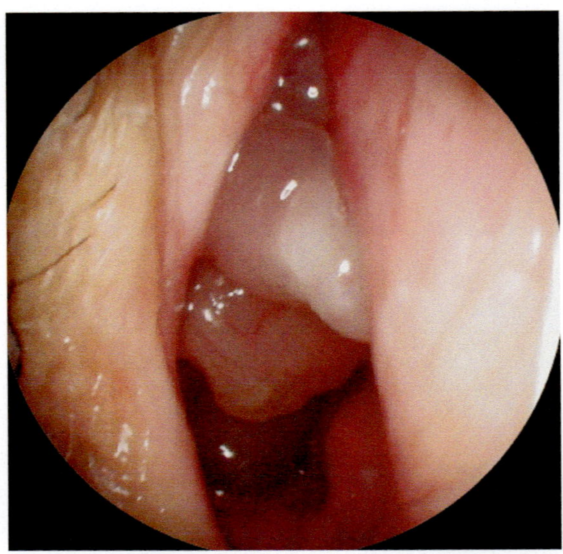

Q. 55. This patient presented with the loss of smell. What is the diagnosis and its subsequent management?

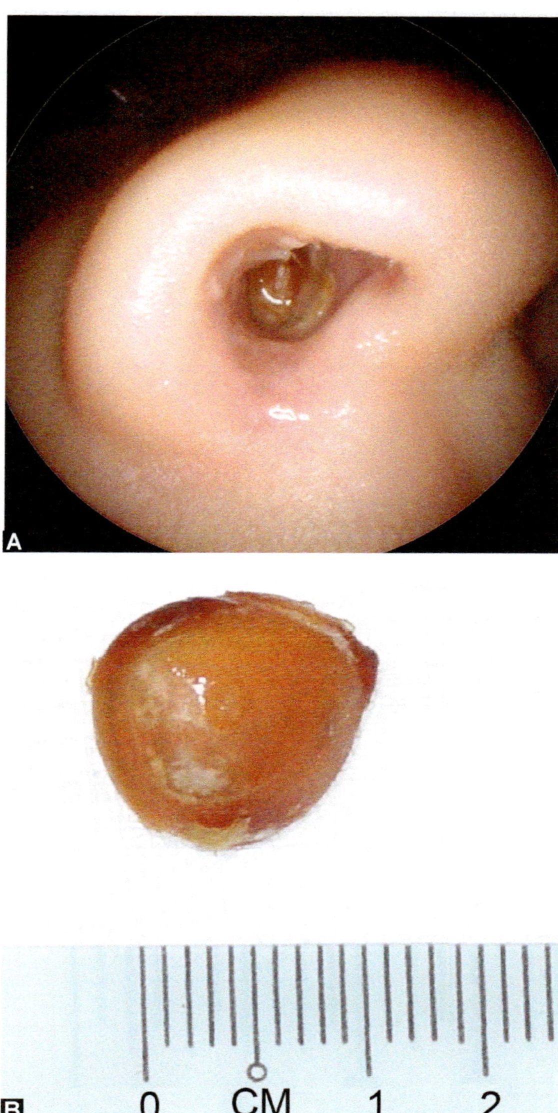

Q. 56. The above child presented with persistent unilateral nasal discharge. How would this child be managed further?

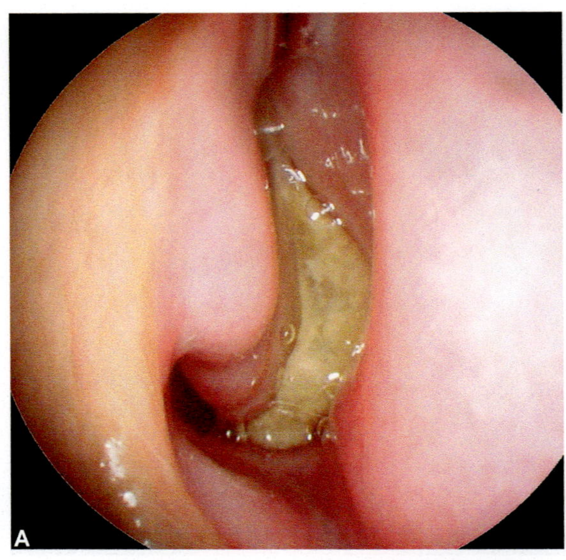

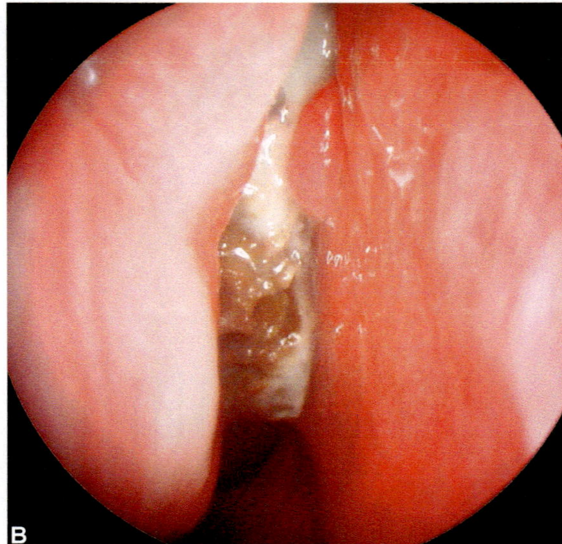

Q. 57. The above patient presented with nasal discharge. Nasal endoscopy followed by suction was performed and the findings were as shown respectively.
What is the likely diagnosis and subsequent management?

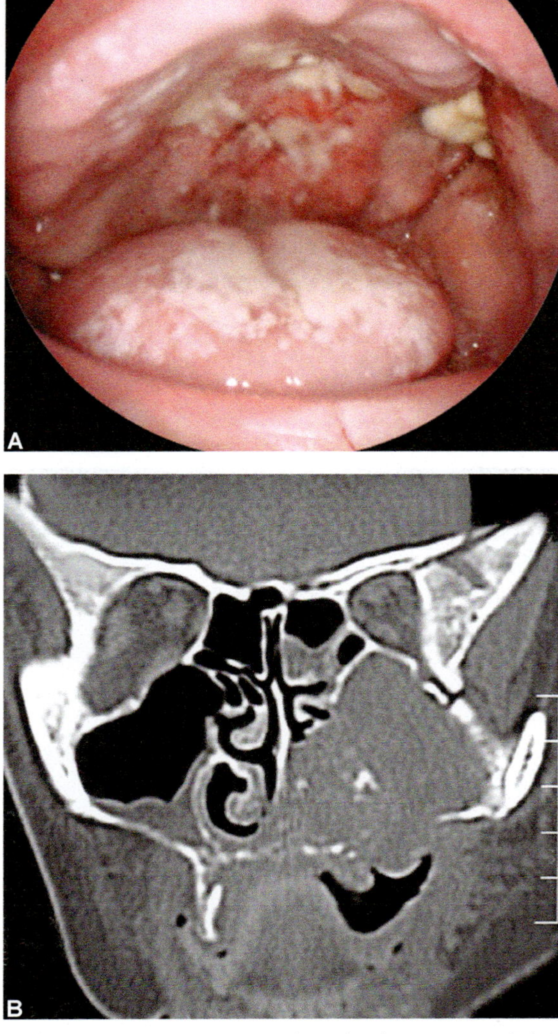

Q. 58. The above patient presented with ulceration of the hard palate.
Computed tomography scan is enclosed.
What is the diagnosis and subsequent management?

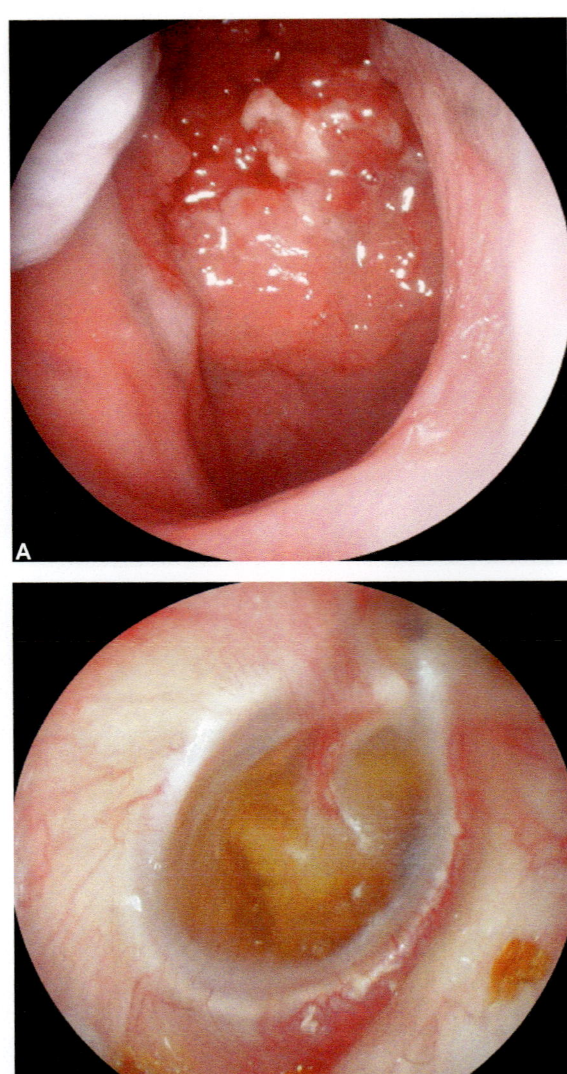

Q. 59. A Chinese gentleman presented with occasional epistaxis and reduced hearing.

a. Describe the findings on endoscopic evaluation.

b. What is the most likely diagnosis and its further management?

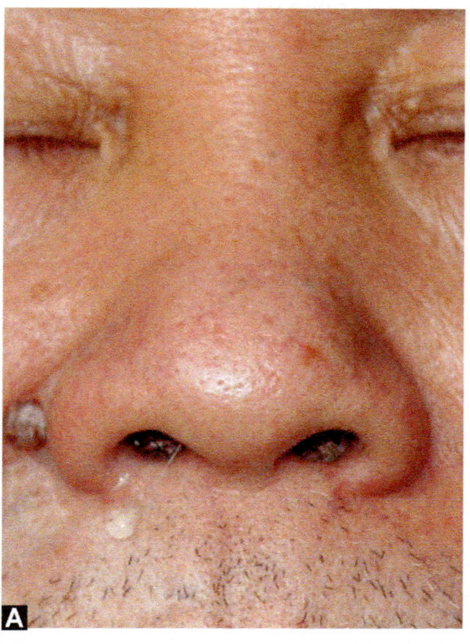

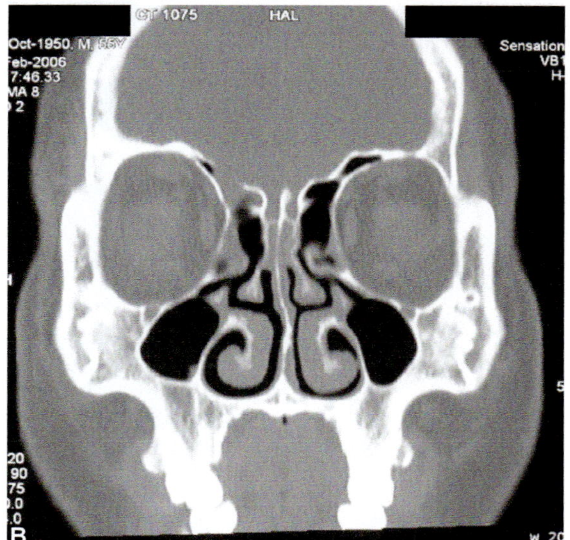

Q. 60. This patient presented with clear nasal drips after an endoscopic nasal procedure.
What is the diagnosis and subsequent management?

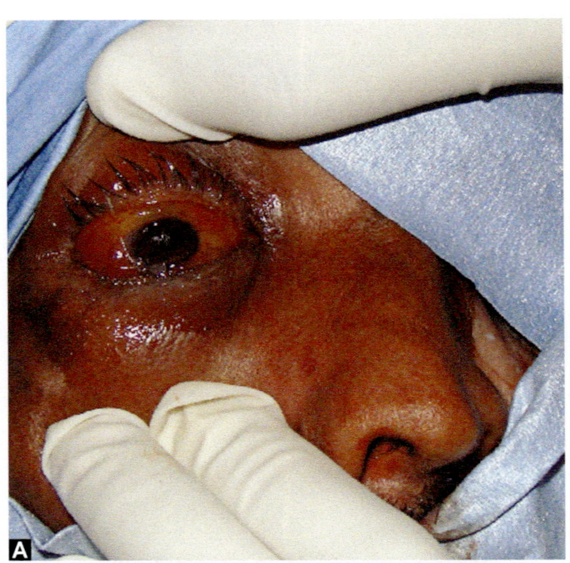

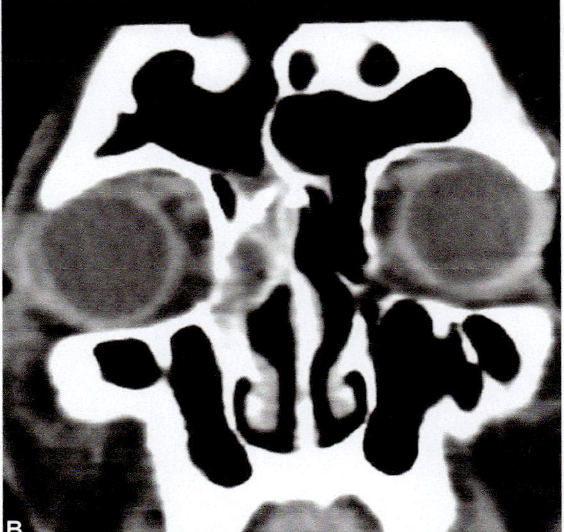

Q. 61. This is a picture of a patient, who developed right eye swelling and reduced eyesight 1 week after he suffered an upper respiratory tract infection.
What is the diagnosis and further management?

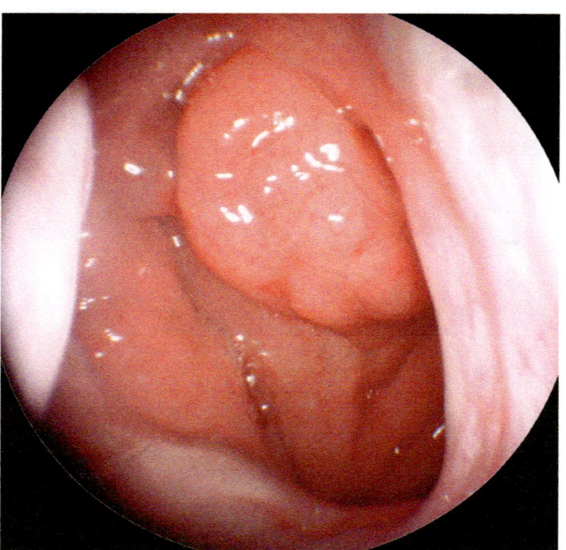

Q. 62. This is an endoscopic view of the nasopharynx in a child. What is seen and how should this case proceed?

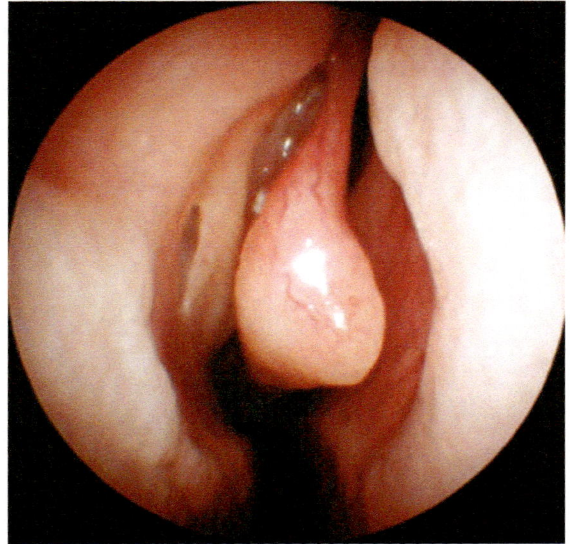

Q. 63. This picture was taken during an endoscopic evaluation of the nasal cavity.

a. Describe the findings.
b. What is the diagnosis and its clinical implications?

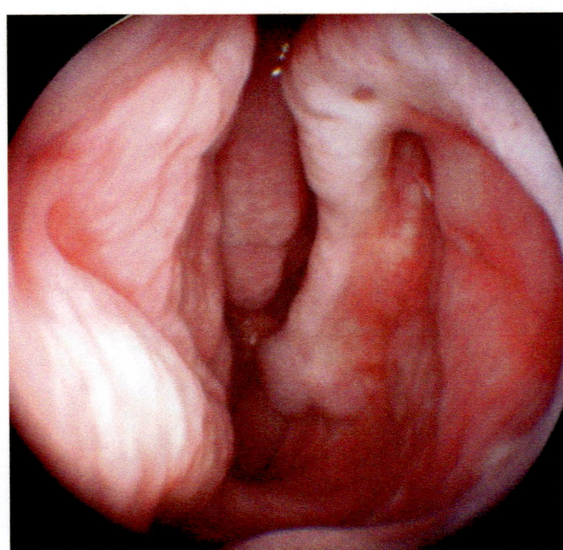

Q. 64. This patient had an operation done to relieve his left nasal obstruction. The endoscopic view is as shown.

a. Describe the findings.
b. What procedure would probably have been done?
c. What precautions are to be considered in this surgery?

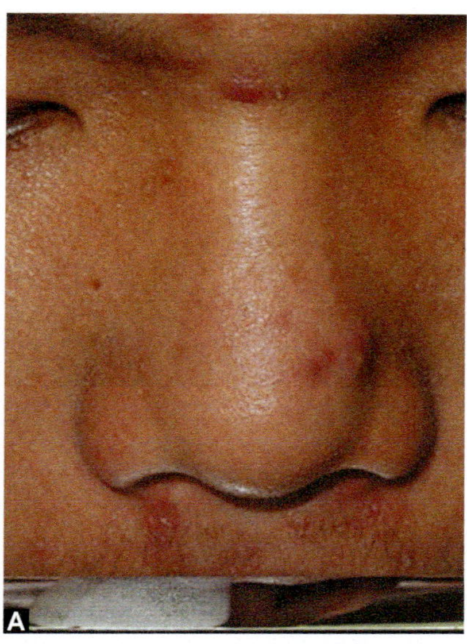
A

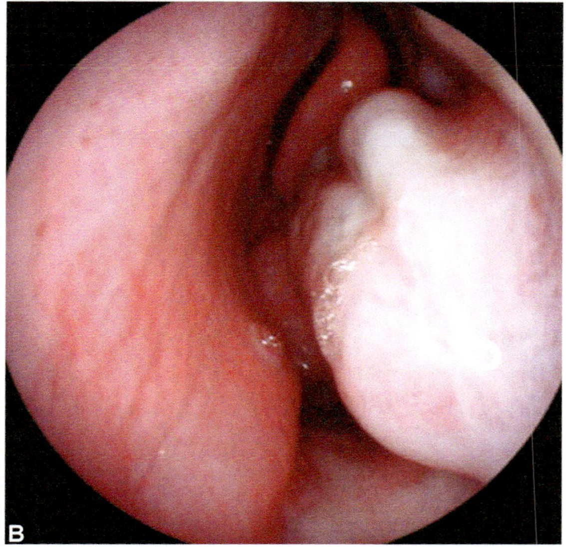
B

Q. 65. A 13-year-old male presented with progressive left nasal obstruction and occasional epistaxis. There were no other ENT complaints of significance.

a. What test is being performed on the patient?
b. Describe the endoscopic findings.
c. What is the most likely diagnosis and its subsequent management?

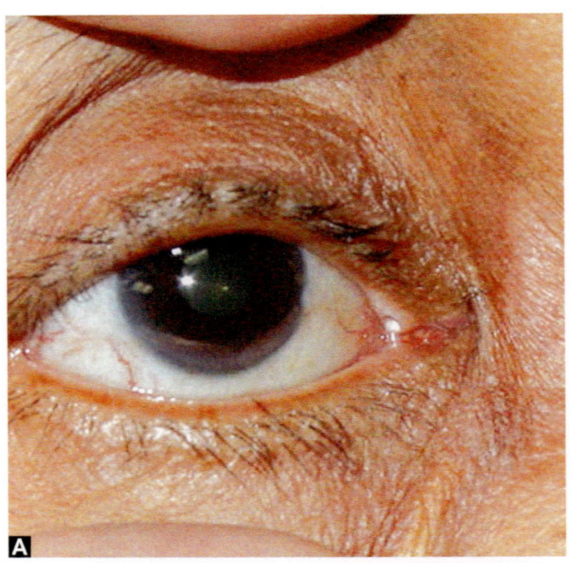

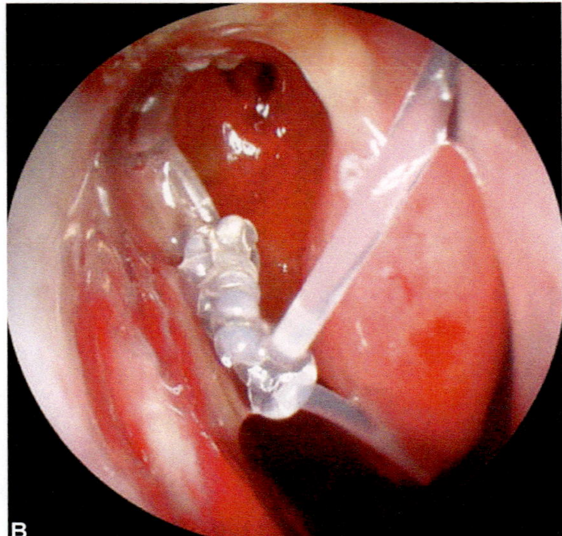

Q. 66. This middle-aged lady had a surgery done to relieve her right watery eye. On follow-up 3 weeks later, her eye was re-examined and nasal endoscopy was performed.

a. Comment on the images shown.
b. What is the subsequent management?

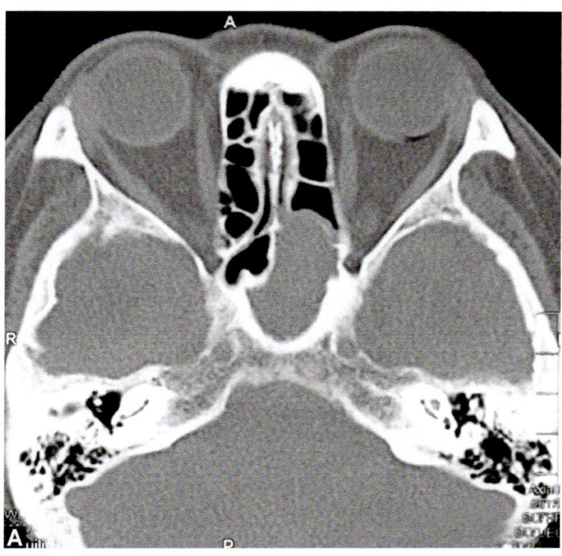

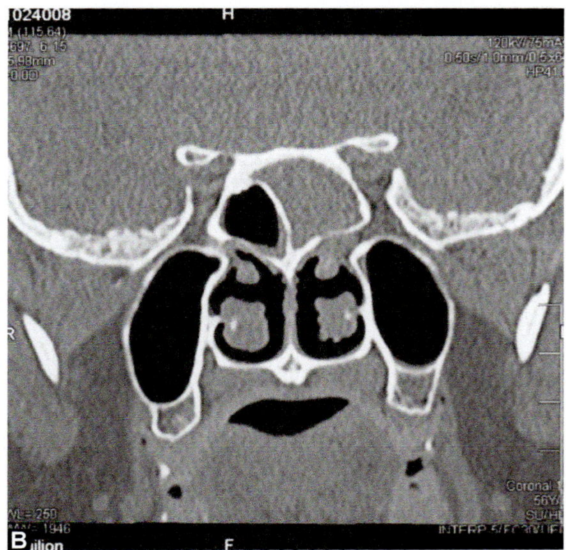

Q. 67. A young gentleman presented with a dull headache for few months duration, which has become persistent at the time of consultation. Nasal endoscopy was performed followed by imaging study.

a. Describe the imaging study findings.
b. What are the possible diagnoses?
c. How would this patient be managed further?

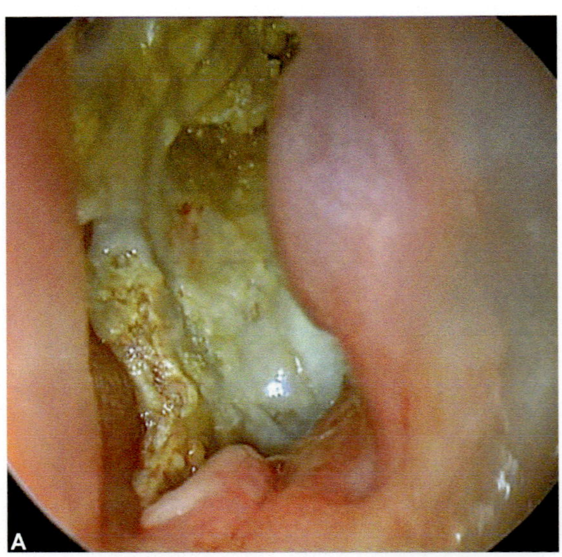

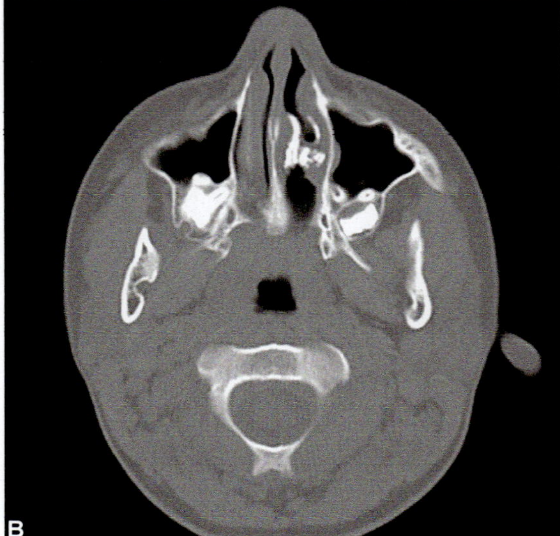

Q. 68. A lady presented with persistent left nasal obstruction for many years, but recently sought consultation due to on-and-off blood-stained nasal discharge, which sometimes becomes smelly. Endoscopic findings were performed followed by imaging study.

a. Describe the nasal findings and correlate it with the radiology image.
b. Give the diagnosis.
c. What is the etiology?
d. How would this patient be treated further?

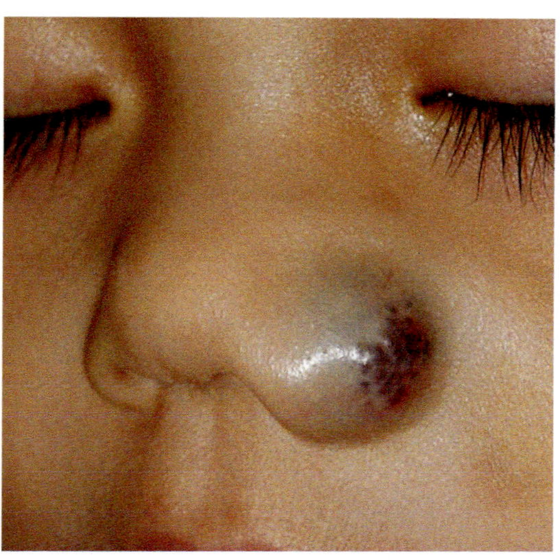

Q. 69. This child was noted to have a slowly enlarging discolored lesion involving her nose. There were no other similar lesions elsewhere and the rest of the ENT examinations were unremarkable.

a. Describe the findings.
b. What is the diagnosis?
c. Outline treatment modalities available for this lesion.

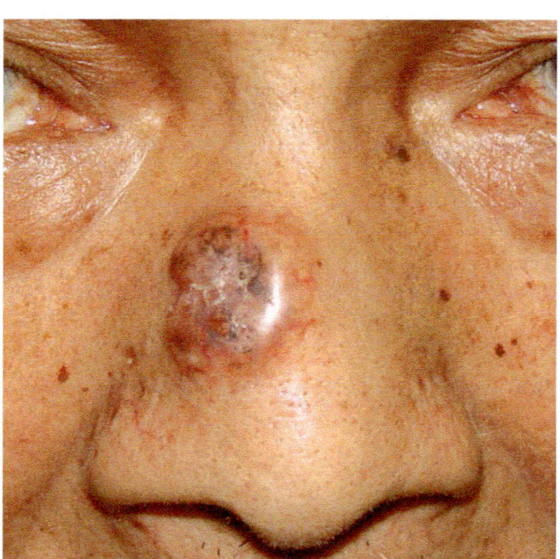

Q. 70. This elderly patient presented with a slowly enlarging swelling involving his nose. There were occasional itchiness but no obvious pain noted.

a. Describe the findings.
b. Give provisional and differential diagnoses.
c. Outline further management of this patient.

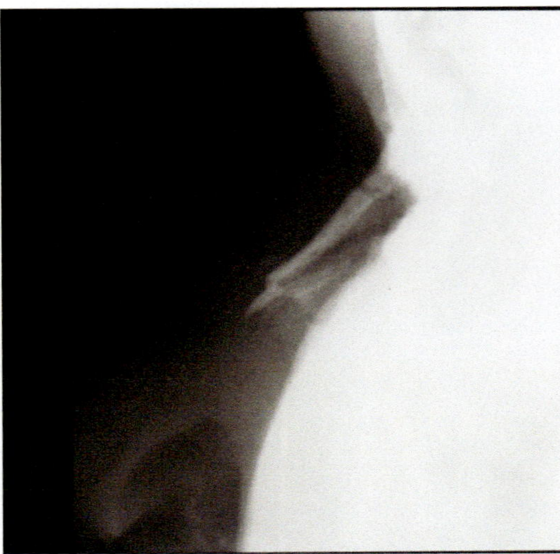

Q. 71. An adult male patient allegedly fell from his bicycle and hit the nose against gravel. There were some epistaxis noted and the bridge of the nose became swollen.

a. Describe the X-ray findings.
b. How would it be fixed?
c. What other lesions should not be missed?

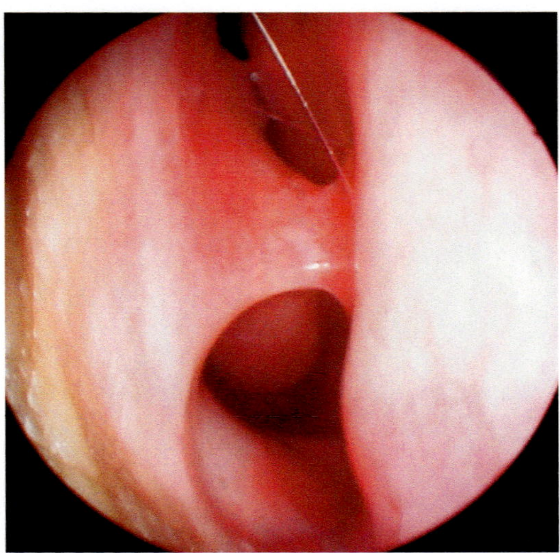

Q. 72. This is an endoscopic image of a patient who had an endoscopic sinus surgery previously. Currently he is well and has no nasal symptom.

a. Describe the findings.
b. What is the diagnosis?
c. How should he be treated?

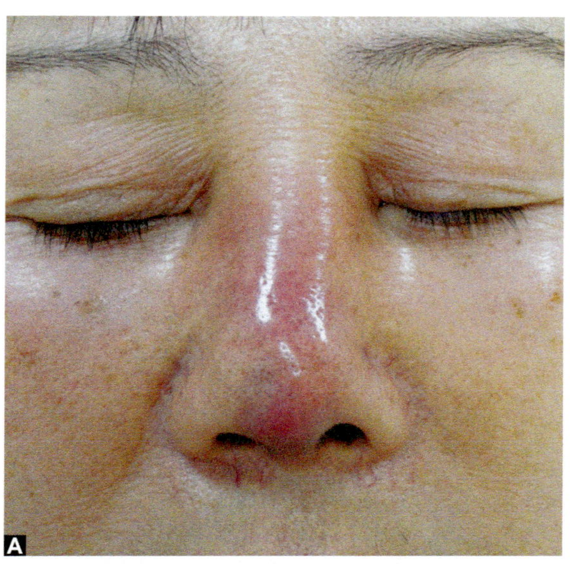

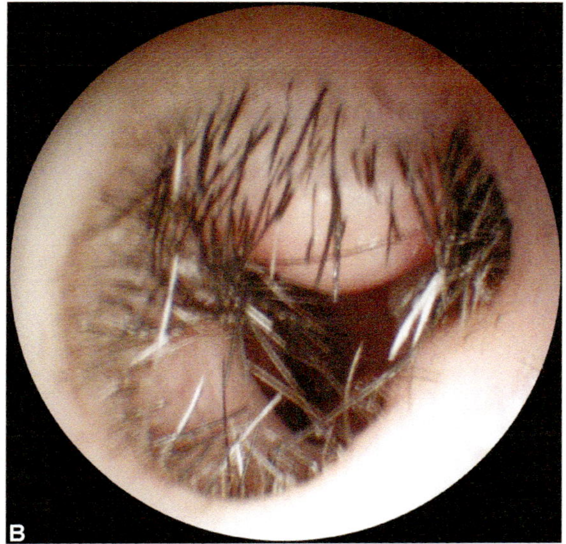

Q. 73. A middle-aged female presented with nasal discoloration and right side nasal blockage for a month duration. She had surgery done previously to make her nose look better. There were no obvious pain, fever, or other nasal symptoms and she is a nondiabetic.

a. Describe the findings of the external nose and right nasal endoscopy.
b. What are the possibilities?
c. How would this patient be treated further?

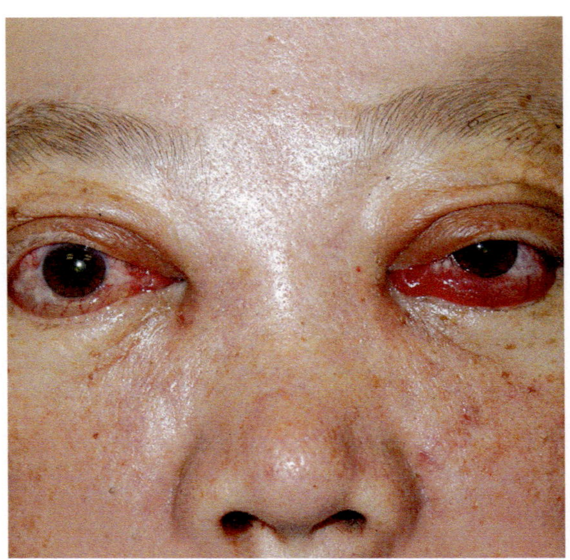

Q. 74. This lady was diagnosed to have nasopharyngeal carcinoma and treated 10 years earlier. She presented now with blurring of vision and examination revealed ophthalmoplegia with visual acuity result of perception to light.

a. Describe the findings.
b. What is the diagnosis?
c. Give the prognosis.

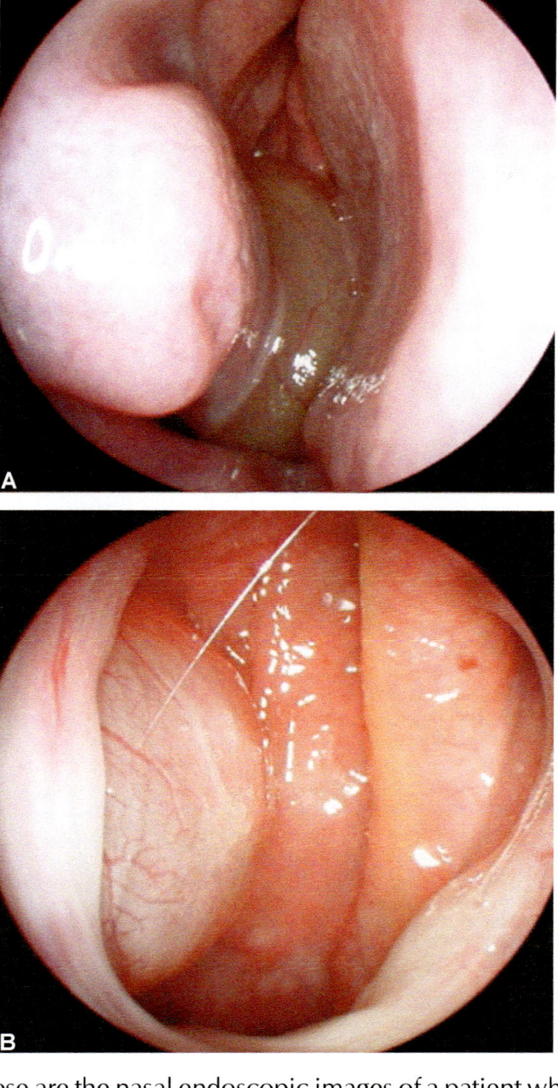

Q. 75. These are the nasal endoscopic images of a patient who presented with unilateral nasal blockage.

a. Describe the findings and give the diagnosis.
b. How would this patient be managed further?

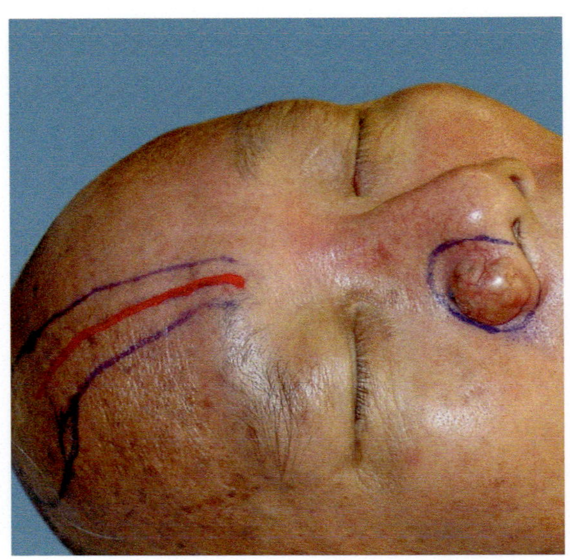

Q. 76. Describe this intraoperative image and discuss the proposed surgery.

Answers

44. a. This is an endoscopic view of the right nasal cavity. The inferior turbinate is seen inferiorly and the middle turbinate appears double with some crustings on its surface. Thus, this could be a bifid turbinate or the lateral structure could be a large uncinate process.

b. The clinical implication is due to the anatomical abnormality that may obstruct the drainage and ventilation of the middle meatus. This will cause disruption of the mucociliary clearance of the sinuses draining into the osteomeatal complex (OMC) and lead to chronic rhinosinusitis. These patients can present with recurrent acute sinusitis, facial heaviness and congestion, postnasal drip and nasal obstruction. Nasal congestion can also lead to mouth breathing and snoring.

c. Management of most anatomical abnormalities usually require surgical intervention if symptomatic as they do not usually resolve with medical therapy. In this case, surgery to clear the middle meatus to establish normal ventilation and drainage of the sinuses will resolve the problems as mentioned.

45. a. This patient is most likely having nasal skin infection. However, underlying vestibulitis should be looked for. In this condition, infection occurs in the nasal vestibule area (the hair-bearing skin of the nasal cavity upto the nasal valve) usually due to minor trauma of the underlying nasal mucosa usually from nose picking. The common organisms implicated are usually *Staphylococcus aureus* and *Streptococcus pyogenes.* The clinical features include indurated skin, swelling, and tenderness of nasal alar or the tip of the nose, with or without sticky nasal discharge, which can be purulent.

b. Severe cases can lead to cellulitis of the surrounding soft tissue which can have serious consequences as this is the dangerous zone of the face. Infection of this area can possibly cause retrograde thrombophlebitis via the ophthalmic vein into the pterygoid plexus and the cavernous sinus. Underlying immunocompromised conditions should be ruled out.

c. Management consists of antibiotics (intravenous in cases of cellulitis) with appropriate analgesics. In chronic cases or recurrent infections, fusidic acid ointment may be applied to the nasal vestibule.

46. a. The nasal examination reveals a deviated nasal septum (DNS) to the left with a compensatory hypertrophy of the right inferior turbinate. The nasal obstruction on the left is further compounded by the fact that the DNS occurs at the nasal valve region. This area, i.e. nasal valve is the narrowest part of the entire upper airway and contributes to at least 50% of the airway resistance.

b. The initial management of this patient consists of a thorough history and clinical examination with endoscopic evaluation to exclude other causes of nasal obstruction. Once the diagnosis is confirmed to be DNS, a septoplasty is warranted to correct the DNS with some form of right turbinate reduction procedure or surgery. It must be explained to the patient that the septal correction would increase the left airway but the right airway could be reduced as compared to preoperatively since the septum will return to the normal place.

47. a. There appears to be a spur arising from the left side of the nasal septum. It is usually a congenital malformation but can also result from trauma. Commonly, the spur is formed at the junction of the bony maxillary crest and the nasal septal cartilage.

b. Patient is usually asymptomatic if it is small, but can experience nasal obstruction if it is large. In some patients, the spur impinges on the middle turbinate causing shooting pain along the nasal bridge. This is known as Sluder's neuralgia, where it is believed to be due to the compression of the ethmoidal nerves.

c. Management of this condition depends on the symptom. It can be left alone if asymptomatic. Persistent symptoms would be an indication of surgical excision of septal spur.

48. a. This is the Little's area of the nose, the area of the anterior portion of the nasal septum most vulnerable to injury particularly during nose picking. It is very vascular supplied by four arteries and commonly bleeds particularly in children. In children, it is believed to be due to the changes in temperature that triggers the bleeding from this area. Prominent subepithelial vessel branches were seen in this patient that would have contributed to the epistaxis events.

b. Management is to complete an endoscopic nasal examination if bleeding persists or becoming recurrent to exclude any other pathology. The prominent vessels can be cauterized. If the septum is deviated, septoplasty could help in addressing the problem.

49. a. This is an endoscopic view of the right nasal cavity that reveals a septal perforation. There appears to be some amount of discharge around it as well. The possible etiologies include postsurgery (iatrogenic), chronic infection (leprosy, tuberculosis, granulomatosis, etc.), or even malignancy. In this case, the perforation is small and the edges appear quite smooth without obvious granulations that are commonly seen in chronic infection or malignancy. Thus, this is most probably an iatrogenic complication.

b. The clinical features range from asymptomatic to whistling sound, bleeding and crustings.

c. The management is directed by the symptom; asymptomatic cases can be left alone. Symptomatic perforations, after excluding infection or malignancy (by biopsy of granulation edges) should be managed with closure by surgery or prosthesis.

50. a. The above patient has a pigmented horizontal crease along dorsum of the nose as well as along either nasolabial folds. This finding is typically found in a patient, who demonstrates the act called "allergic salute".

b. It is due to allergic rhinitis, where frequent wiping or rubbing (usually upward) of the nose that is associated with rhinitis causes crease formation along its dorsum with variable degree of pigmentation. The management is to treat the underlying cause as most patients do not even notice the crease.

51. a. The image is of the right nasal cavity. It shows a mild deviation of the upper nasal septum to the right with inferior turbinate hypertrophy that is compromising the right nasal airway.

b. The etiology of the inferior turbinate hypertrophy is multifactorial ranging from compensatory enlargement secondary to nasal septum deviation to allergy, vasomotor rhinitis, hormonal changes and chronic infection.

c. The management consists of determining the initial causative factor and treating the underlying cause if possible. Following which, a course of nasal corticosteroids and/or antihistamine with or without decongestants can be used. If it persisted despite this treatment, surgical intervention can be considered, ranging from surface cautery and submucous diathermy to the more invasive turbinoplasty or even turbinectomy.

52. a. Image appears to be an endoscopic view of the left nasal cavity that reveals a mucopurulent discharge from the left middle meatus. This is the characteristic of acute maxillary sinusitis. The presence of pus discharging from the middle meatus is a good indicator as it suggests the maxilla is draining and the ostium is patent. Acute maxillary sinusitis, that is not draining tends to present with acute facial pain and in severe cases can cause complications, e.g. to the orbit. The sinus X-ray shows opacity of the left maxilla that is consistent with sinusitis. It is important to note that a unilateral recurrent maxillary sinusitis could be due to dental infections as the upper molars are embedded into the floor of the maxilla.

b. The management consists of antibiotics, decongestants and analgesics in the initial stages. Recurrent episodes would indicate an underlying dental pathology or chronic rhinosinusitis, which should be treated accordingly.

53. a. The endoscopic view of the right nasal cavity reveals a large middle turbinate and the computed tomography (CT) scan confirms the clinical impression of concha bullosa. This is defined as a pneumatized middle turbinate or simply the presence of air cell within the middle concha. It is probably one of the most common anatomical anomalies seen in the nasal cavity. Concha bullosa may remain asymptomatic and only be found incidentally on nasal endoscopy. However, it can block the OMC, which would lead to reduced ventilation and drainage of the sinuses; thus, predispose to recurrent acute sinusitis or chronic rhinosinusitis.

b. The treatment is usually surgical as most anatomical abnormalities do not respond to medical therapy. The CT scan shows quite clearly the large pneumatized middle turbinate and DNS to the left. Thus, the pneumatization could be a compensatory mechanism. The OMC appears to be compromised in the CT scan, which would have predisposed this patient to recurrent sinusitis.

54. The right nasal cavity appears to be filled with a fleshy vascular mass medial to the inferior turbinate. The CT scan reveals opacity of the right nasal cavity, OMC, and ethmoid sinuses with mucosal thickening of the maxillary sinuses. There is no bone erosion or destruction noted, thus this tumor is probably benign. Management includes a thorough history, clinical examination with nasal endoscope and a biopsy to confirm the histological diagnosis. A unilateral nasal mass without bony destruction is most likely to be an inverted papilloma or antrochoanal polyp. The absence of opacity in the maxillary sinus in the CT scan excludes antrochoanal polyp.

55. There appears to be multiple smooth, glistening swellings in the right nasal cavity, which are typical of nasal polyps. They usually present with nasal obstruction and loss of smell. Facial pain and discomfort is not common, which helps to differentiate this condition from chronic rhinosinusitis. If they are bilateral, they are ethmoidal polyps, while antrochoanal polyps are unilateral in nature. The management consists of an initial biopsy to confirm the diagnosis and followed by nasal corticosteroid spray or even oral steroids in severe cases. In cases where the obstruction is complete, surgical modality may be employed.

56. There appears to be a brownish mass in the right nostril, which turned out to be a fruit seed (foreign body). This diagnosis must always be considered in a child with persistent unilateral nasal discharge. The foreign body can be removed in the clinic with the child wrapped or held tightly by his/her parent with the use of right instrument. Failure of which, removal under general anesthesia (GA) would be required.

57. The nasal cavity appears to be filled with slate-brown material covered with purulent discharge. This finding is usually seen in patient with fungal sinusitis and would require a thorough nasal endoscopy, removal of infected material, and mucosal biopsy. Secretion should be sent to look for fungal hyphae. Once the diagnosis is confirmed, CT scan of the paranasal sinuses (PNS) is ordered to assess the extent of the disease. Endoscopy-assisted surgical debridement can be performed and in cases of invasive fungal sinusitis in immunocompromised patient, systemic antifungal may be required.

58. The ulceration appears located at the posterior aspect of hard palate and its junction with the soft palate. It has an exophytic edge with marked areas of granulations. The dorsal surface of the tongue is covered with white material, probably an oral thrush. The CT scan showed complete opacification of the left maxillary cavity with erosions involving its floor and the lateral nasal wall. The inferior turbinate and part of the nasal septum were destroyed as well. Bony erosion and destruction usually indicate a malignancy. In this case, the diagnosis is most likely carcinoma (CA) of maxilla, which would have started from its floor. Management consists of confirming the diagnosis with histopathological examination (HPE) and investigation to exclude distant metastasis. Total maxillectomy, followed by radiotherapy or chemotherapy as advised by the oncologist would be the recommended scheme of treatment.

59. a. The nasendoscopic view of the nasopharynx reveals an ulcerofungating mass involving the fossa of Rosenmüller (FOR) and the posterior wall of nasopharynx. The right otoendoscopic view reveals a retracted tympanic membrane with yellowish fluid in the middle ear (serous otitis media, middle ear effusion, glue ear).

b. These are typical findings of nasopharyngeal carcinoma, which is a common malignancy especially among the Chinese. It is believed to be due to Epstein-Barr virus, although the triggering factor is still unknown. The obstructive effect of the tumor on the Eustachian tube (ET) causes a negative middle ear pressure and accumulation of fluid in the middle ear space. Once the diagnosis is confirmed histologically (to exclude lymphoma especially in WHO type III), imaging modalities (computed tomography, magnetic resonance imaging, positron emission tomography scan, bone scan, ultrasound of liver) are used to determine its local extent, presence of distant metastasis, and help in staging of the disease. Treatment options include radiotherapy with or without chemotherapy depending on the stage. Myringotomy and grommet insertion will alleviate hearing loss while the tumor is being treated.

60. This is a bone window view of coronal cut CT scan of the PNS. There is a defect of the right fovea ethmoidalis with herniation of intracranial content into the nasal cavity. A clear drip after an endoscopic sinus surgery should always be presumed a cerebrospinal fluid (CSF) leak. Initial management includes confirming the fluid as CSF (beta-transferrin test) and investigation to locate the site of leak. If the defect is large, CT scan would be able to demonstrate the exact location. However, smaller defect may be missed. Sometimes, a fluorescein dye is used intrathecally to identify the leak. If the leak persists (most small leaks heal spontaneously), an endoscopic repair may be carried out. The choice of graft material for repair ranges from septal mucoperichondrial graft to fascia lata. In some cases, lumbar drain is inserted by some surgeons.

61. The picture shows an orbital complication of acute sinusitis. The right eye appears swollen with its conjunctiva suffused and edematous which also seem to be pushed inferiorly. This is usually due to subperiosteal cellulitis, which complicates to abscess formation as a result of extension of pus from the ethmoid sinusitis breaching the lamina papyracea. The CT scan illustrates this well on the right side, where there is opacity of the right ethmoid with collection of pus between the medial wall of the orbit and the eyeball itself. This causes the orbit to be compressed and may eventually result in vision loss; thus this is an emergency. The patient needs to be admitted and started on intravenous antibiotics. An ophthalmology consultation should be obtained and if there is vision reduction or the presence of sub-perichondrial abscess in the CT scan, the pus should be drained via open Lynch-Howarth incision or endoscopically according to the surgeon's experience.

62. The image shows a moderate size adenoid tissue along the roof and posterior wall of nasopharynx. Adenoids are normal in children especially between the ages of 6–8 years. Most of them are asymptomatic and can be left alone. Enlarged adenoids can obstruct the nasopharynx and ET leading to mouth breathing, snoring, apnea and glue ear. Adenoids should only be removed if they are large and symptomatic. Nasopharyngeal CA on the other hand, originates usually from the lateral aspect of nasopharynx (FOR) and rarely seen in children.

63. a. This is an image of the right middle meatus. It shows an oval-shaped opening in front of the outline of the uncinate process. There is no polyp or mucopus noted and the OMC area appears free from any obstruction.

b. An accessory maxillary ostium. This ostium is usually located more anteriorly and found in front of the uncinate process (it can be multiple) as compared to the natural ostium, which is sited higher and posterior to it; thus unusual to be seen directly on viewing using 0° endoscope. It can be the passage for an antrochoanal polyp as it exits from the antrum before heading posteriorly toward the choana. Physiologically, mucociliary function and drainage of the maxillary sinus is directed toward natural ostium. If an ostia is noted without the uncinate being removed, then it is almost always an accessory ostia.

64. a. Image showed absence of entire left inferior turbinate with the exception of its posterior end. Mucous membrane covering the inferior concha remains. Opening of the nasolacrimal duct is clearly seen and appears patent. There is a furrow and buckling of the septum toward the opposite site likely caused by DNS. The middle turbinate and nasopharynx can be seen.

b. Subtotal inferior turbinate trimming or turbinectomy. It was probably done to relieve persistent nasal obstruction caused by compensatory inferior turbinate hypertrophy secondary to the DNS.

c. Perioperative bleeding can be significant. This is especially so when its posterior end is encroached upon (branches from sphenopalatine vessels). Thus, postoperative nasal packing is necessary. This procedure should not be performed in cold countries to avoid crustings and possible development of secondary atrophic rhinitis. Presently, alternative procedures are available ranging from superficial cautery, radiofrequency, powered instruments, or even laser. These treatment options need to be discussed with the patient and the procedure chosen should cause minimal morbidity with lasting effects.

65. a. This patient appears to have a totally reduced airway on the left side as demonstrated by the cold spatula test.

b. Endoscopic nasal examination revealed a mass along the floor of the left nasal cavity below the middle turbinate.

c. A history of recurrent epistaxis in a boy should alert the clinician to the diagnosis of angiofibroma and above-mentioned findings would clinically confirm angiofibroma. Management consists of confirming the diagnosis with a CT contrast, where a blush is noted due to the vascularity of the lesion. The tumor extents are noted as it can involve the pterygopalatine fossa or even extend intracranially. Treatment is usually by surgical excision either endoscopically or via open traditional approach after an embolization procedure.

66. a. The images reveal evidence of a post endoscopic dacryocystorhinostomy (DCR), which is usually performed for patients with epiphora. The ophthalmologists usually flush the canaliculi and if this fails to relieve epiphora, then the option of DCR is offered to the patient. A silicon tune (O'Donoghue or Jones) is inserted into both the upper and lower canaliculi and delivered into the lacrimal sac and secured intranasally.

b. The tube is kept for an average of 3 months and then removed in an outpatient setting. In our experience, a success rate of 94% can be achieved this way.

67. a. The PNS CT scan shows the left sphenoid sinuses filled with soft tissue density mass or fluid that displaces the anterior sphenoidal wall. The bony margins are thickened and ossified indicating the possibility of osteogenesis.

b. The possible diagnosis includes left sphenoidal mucocele, polyps, sinusitis, fungal sinusitis or sphenoidal tumor.

c. The patient will require an endoscopic examination, especially of the sphenoid-ethmoid complex. The management would surgically intervene, where sphenoidotomy will be required to excise and examine the origin of the mass. Biopsy is mandatory.

68. a. The nasal endoscopic examination reveals a crusted lesion covered with mucopus in the left nasal cavity. The PNS CT scan reveals left nasal cavity mass with calcification.

b. The diagnosis is left nasal cavity rhinolith.

c. The etiology is the formation of calculi in the nasal cavity, which usually occurs around the nucleus of a small exogenous foreign body, blood clot or impissated secretion by slow deposition of calcium and magnesium salts.

d. The patient should undergo removal of the rhinolith under sedation. Later, she needs to perform regular nasal douche and take antibiotics to cover infection.

69. a. The image reveals a child's face with a bluish discoloration noted at the left alar of the nose.

b. The most likely diagnosis is left alar hemangioma or arteriovenous malformation.

c. Most of this lesion can be treated conservatively as the lesion will regress with age. If there is no regression, we can consider medical treatment like propranolol or give option of surgery to excise the lesion.

70. a. This photo shows a middle-aged gentleman's face with a mid nasal mass located at its right side wall encroaching the midline. The edges appeared elevated with early formation of ulcer evident by shallow central slope and scab formation.

b. The provisional diagnosis is basal cell carcinoma (BCC) and the differential diagnoses are squamous cell CA and verrucous CA.

c. This patient needs to undergo a wide local excision of the lesion with clear margin. Later, a rotation flap can be harvested to cover the excised skin.

71. a. The X-ray shows a nasal bone fracture.

b. The fracture can be fixed with closed reduction either under local anesthesia infiltration or under GA.

c. Other lesions that should not be missed include septal hematoma, craniofacial fractures, and intracranial injuries.

72. a. This endoscopic image shows a synechia of right nasal cavity with an adjoining adhesion between right nasal wall and septum.

b. The diagnosis is post endoscopic sinus surgery synechiae.

c. He can be treated either conservatively or surgically. As he is well and without nasal symptoms, wait and see policy can be applied here. However, if the nasal symptom occurs and proved related to this scar tissue, its excision is then recommended with temporary insertion of intranasal splint for about a week.

73. a. The left photo shows red and swollen external nose with deviation of dorsum of the nose and the right nasal endoscopic view shows a swelling involving the superior part of the vestibule.

b. The possibilities are extrusion of implant in the nose, and cellulitis of the external nose, as well as foreign body granulomatous reaction.

c. This patient should be admitted and start parental antibiotics. The extruded and infected implant should be removed and immediate surrounding tissue biopsied.

74. a. This lady has bilateral conjunctival chemosis, lids edema and redness of the eyes.

b. The possible diagnosis is cavernous sinus thrombosis resulting from direct upward spread of the recurrence tumor and invasions of the cavernous sinus.

c. The prognosis is poor.

75. a. The nasal endoscopic images show a glistening polypoidal mass with a smooth surface in right nasal cavity and extending posteriorly to the nasopharynx. The most likely diagnosis will be antrochoanal polyp.

b. A PNS CT scan should be ordered to assess the origin and extent of the polypoidal mass. Later, the mass should be removed and sent for HPE.

76. This image shows a gentleman with right nasal alar skin lesion (likely BCC) with planning of glabellar/forehead rotation skin flap. This flap will be excised and sutured once taken well by the recipient site and viable.

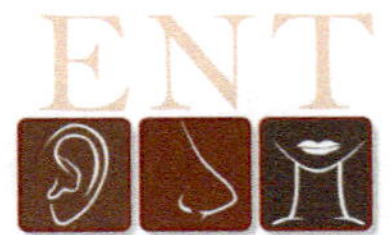

3 HEAD AND NECK

Questions

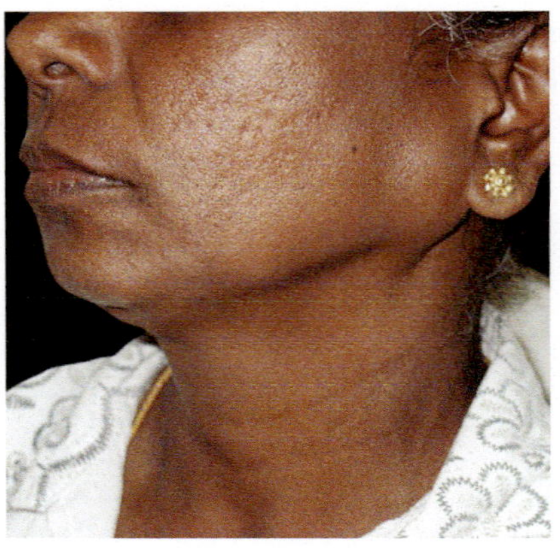

Q. 77. This patient developed a gradual painless swelling in front of the left ear. She did not have any other complaints.

a. What are the possible diagnoses?

b. What is the subsequent management?

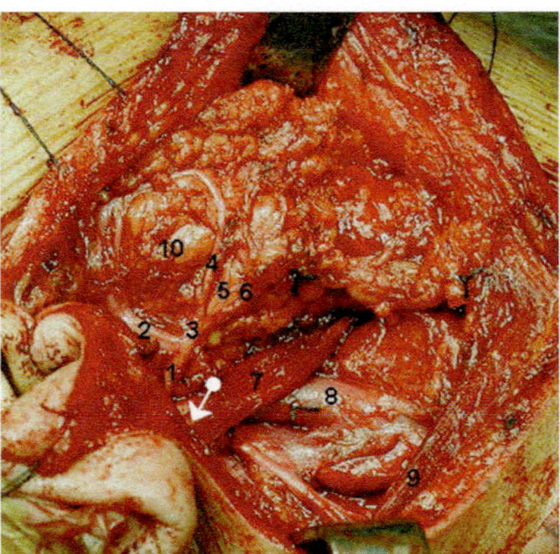

Q. 78. This patient had superficial parotidectomy performed.

a. Name the structures as numbered.

b. What are the landmarks that can be used to identify facial nerve intraoperatively?

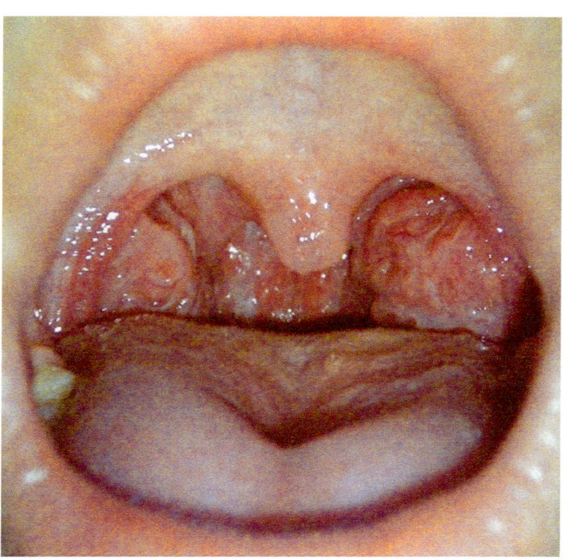

Q. 79. This patient complained of recurrent sore throat associated with fever. What is the diagnosis and subsequent management?

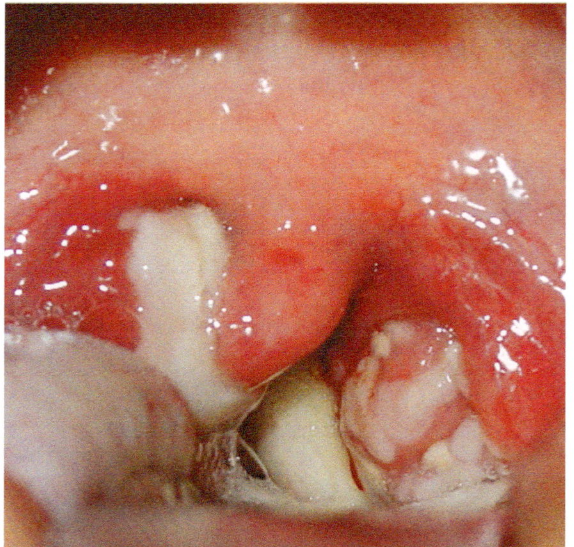

Q. 80. This patient presented with high fever for 3 days duration, associated with severe odynophagia and inability to tolerate orally. Neck examination revealed multiple tender cervical lymphadenopathy.

a. Describe the findings on throat examination.
b. What is the diagnosis?
c. What complications can occur?
d. How would this patient be managed?

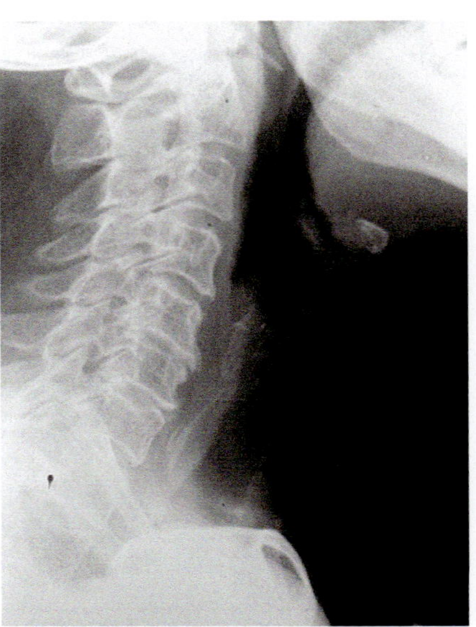

Q. 81. An elderly lady was admitted with odynophagia after a meal. Examination revealed pooling of saliva in the hypopharynx, upon which a lateral neck X-ray was ordered.

a. Describe the X-ray findings.
b. What is the subsequent management?

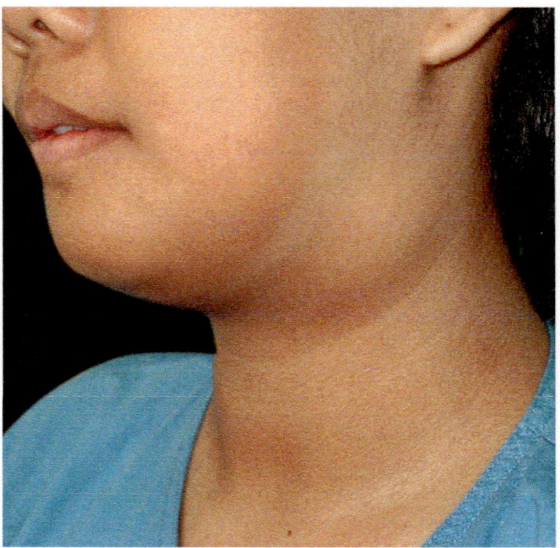

Q. 82. This 14-year-old girl complained of slow growing painless swelling over left anterior triangle of the neck. Computed tomography scan showed a well-defined hypodense cystic lesion.

List the possible etiologies and its subsequent management.

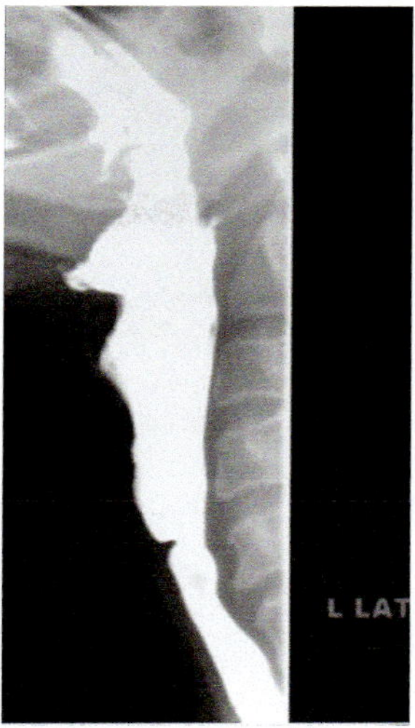

Q. 83. This 40-year-old lady presented with dysphagia to solid foods since past 2 years. No loss of appetite or weight loss was noted. Investigations showed Hb: 84.7 g/l, MCV: 72 fl, MCH: 21.1 pg, MCHC: 294 g/l, serum ferritin: 7.2 μg/l, serum iron: 2.35 μmol/l.

a. Describe the barium swallow findings.
b. What is the diagnosis?
c. How would this patient be managed further?

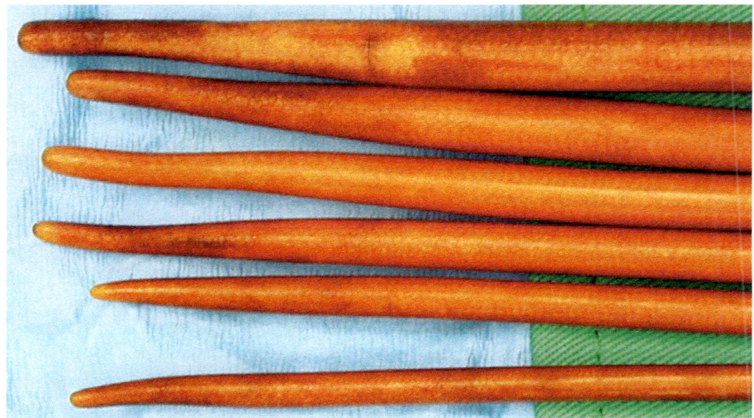

Q. 84. What is shown and what are its indications?

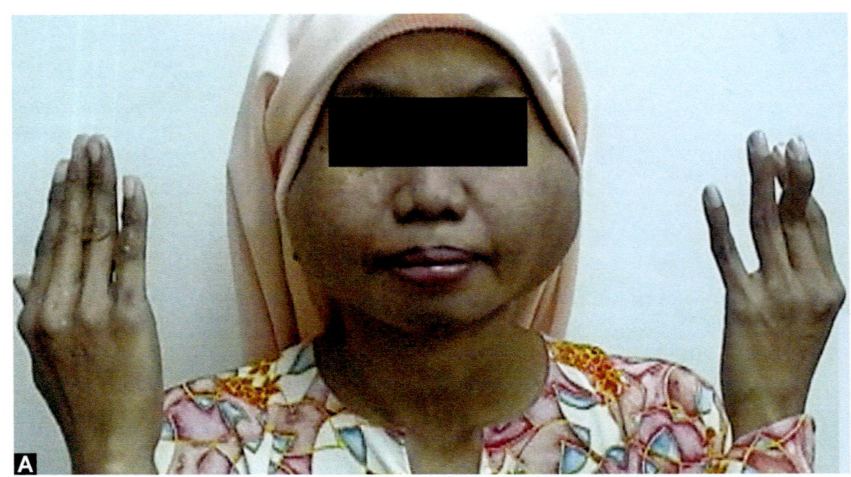

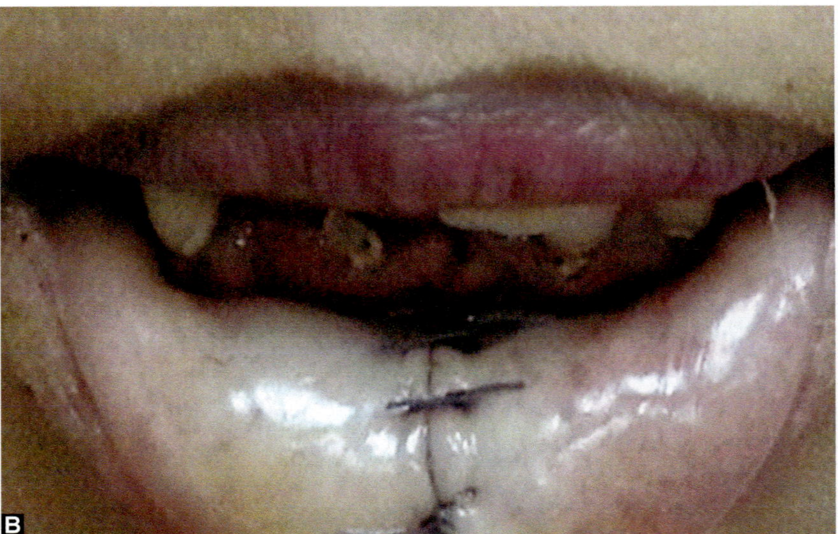

Q. 85. This patient presented in the ENT clinic with complaints of bilateral parotid swellings and hand problems.

a. What is the diagnosis?
b. Why do these patients present with the ENT clinic?
c. What does the picture of her lips indicate?

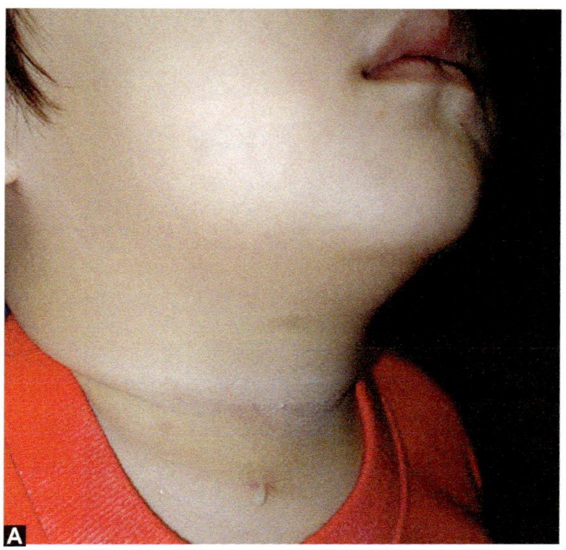

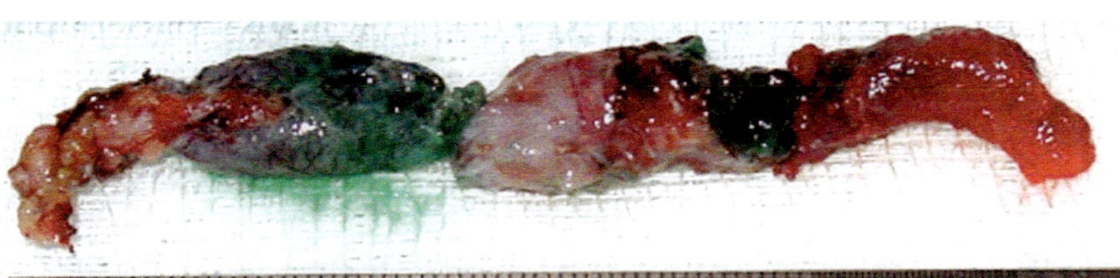

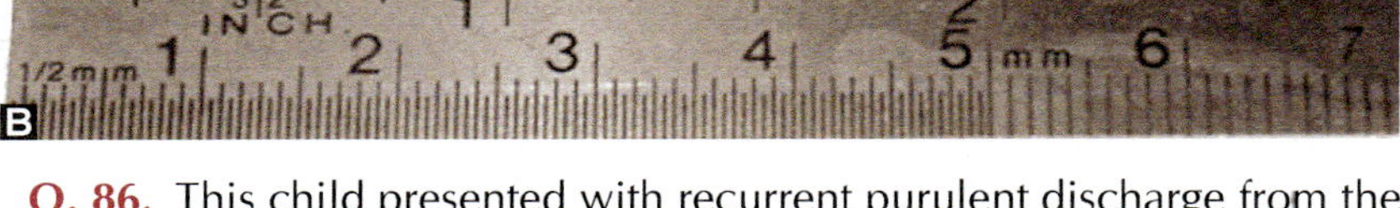

Q. 86. This child presented with recurrent purulent discharge from the lower neck near midline. Neck exploration was performed after the infection settled and specimen as shown was obtained.

a. What is the diagnosis?

b. Where else in head and other areas similar lesion can occur?

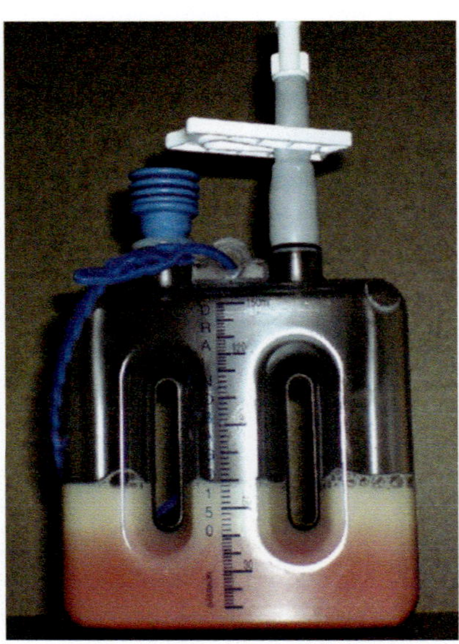

Q. 87. Left radical neck dissection was performed in a patient with metastatic cervical lymphadenopathy from carcinoma of larynx. Redivac drain and collection bottle is shown above.

a. What is the likely diagnosis?
b. How would this patient be managed further?

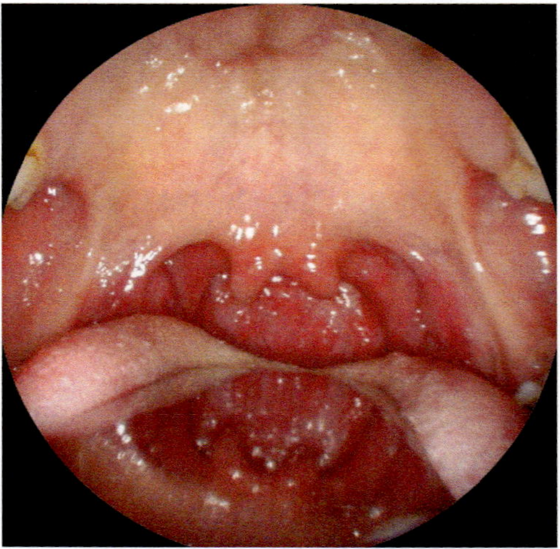

Q. 88. This patient presented with a reduced hearing and mild nasal speech. Oropharyngeal findings were as shown.

a. What is the diagnosis?
b. What is the likely cause of his reduced hearing in relation to this finding?
c. How would this patient be managed further?

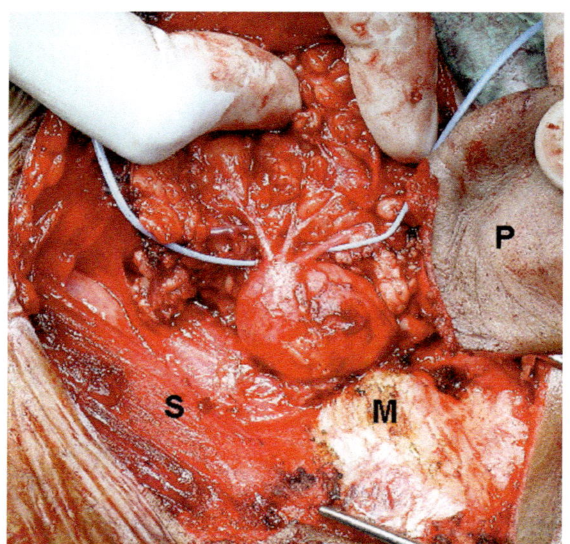

Q. 89. This is an intraoperative finding during a routine surgery for a parotid swelling.
What is the diagnosis and the subsequent management?

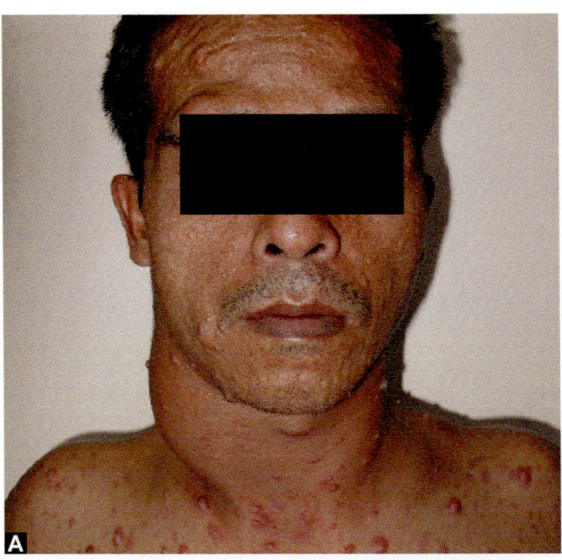

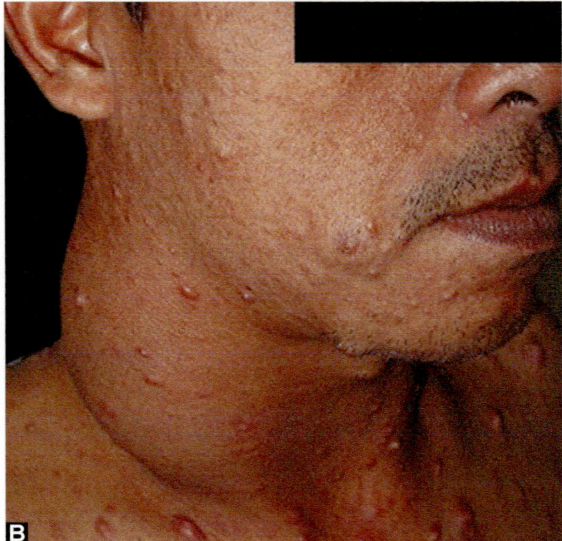

Q. 90. This patient presented with multiple firm swellings of various sizes involving the skin of the whole body. He also has a bigger neck lump on the right side of his neck.

a. What is the diagnosis?
b. What are the other manifestations of the disease in the head and the neck area?

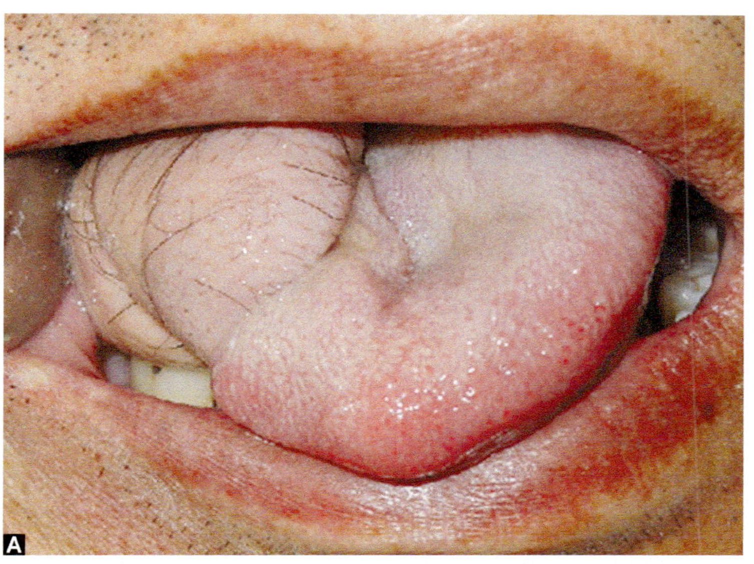

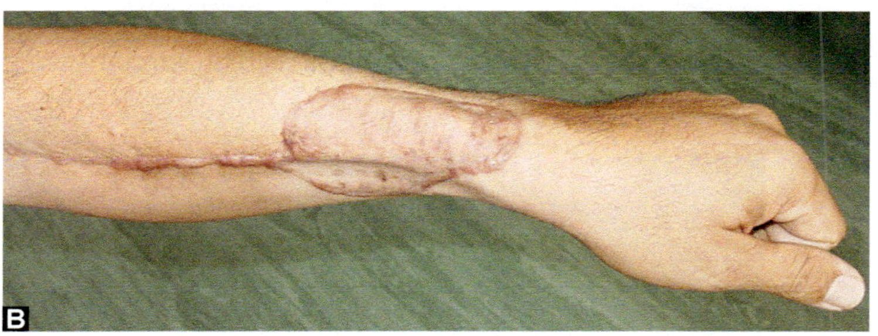

Q. 91. The above patient had an operation for a lesion involving the right side of his tongue. On follow-up, oral cavity and forearm examinations revealed the above findings.

a. With what condition this patient would have suffered prior to the operation?
b. What operation was performed and its indication?
c. What other options are available for similar lesion?

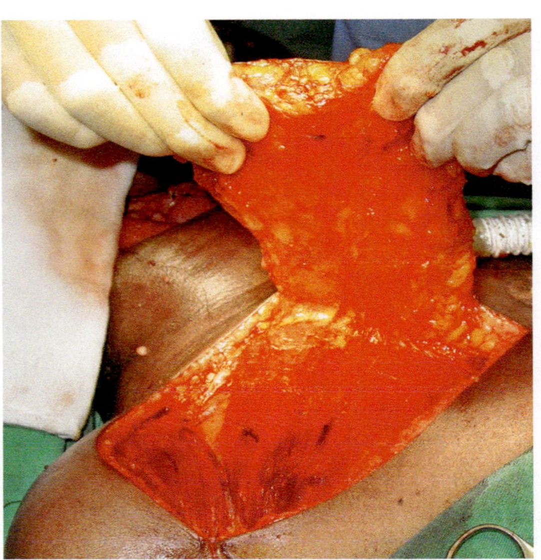

Q. 92. This picture was taken during an oncologic surgery. What is being performed and under which circumstance the procedure is necessary?

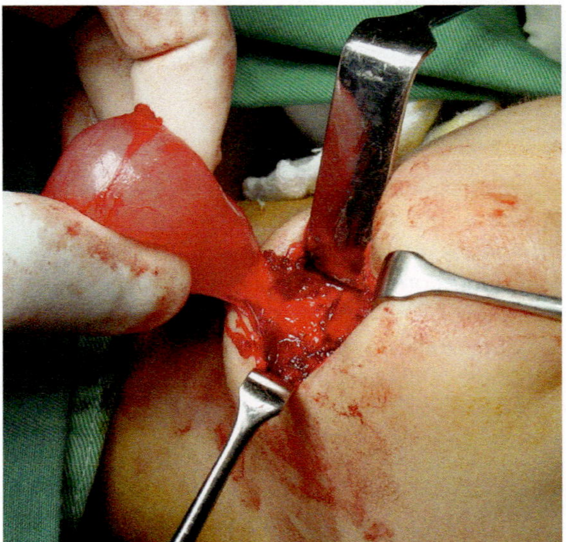

Q. 93. This is an intraoperative image of a child, who presented earlier with a painless central neck swelling.

a. What is shown?
b. Give the diagnosis.
c. Briefly describe the operative procedure.

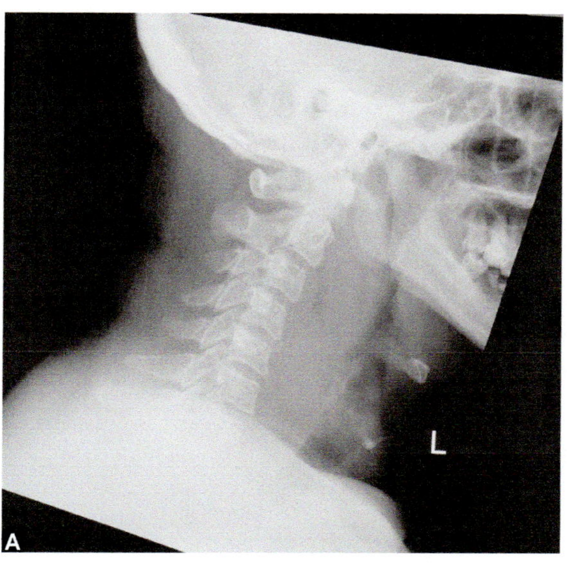

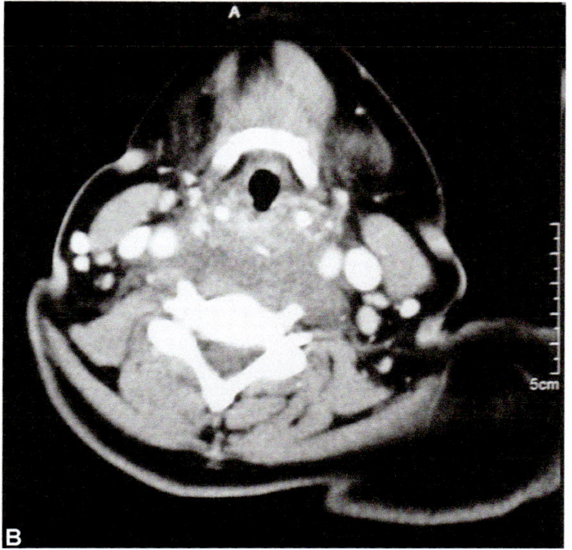

Q. 94. A 54-year-old female with noninsulin dependent diabetes mellitus presented with severe odynophagia and fever since 4 days prior to admission. She denied having difficulty in breathing or stridor. On examination, she appeared dehydrated and the neck was swollen. Random blood sugar test showed reading of 18 mmol/l. Imaging studies were ordered as shown.

a. Describe the findings of both radiological images.
b. What is the likely diagnosis?
c. Outline further management of this patient.

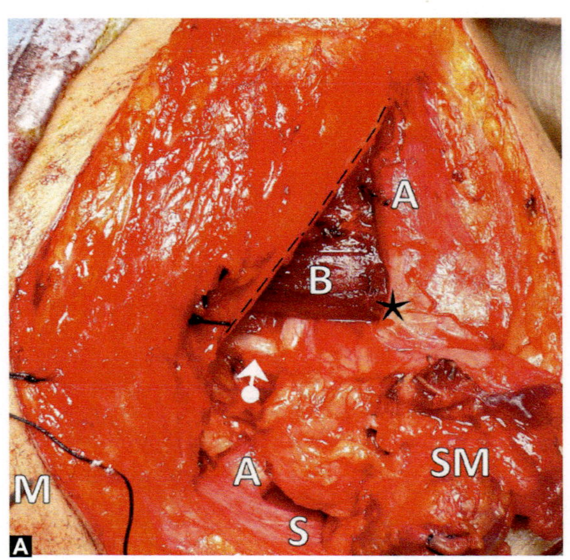

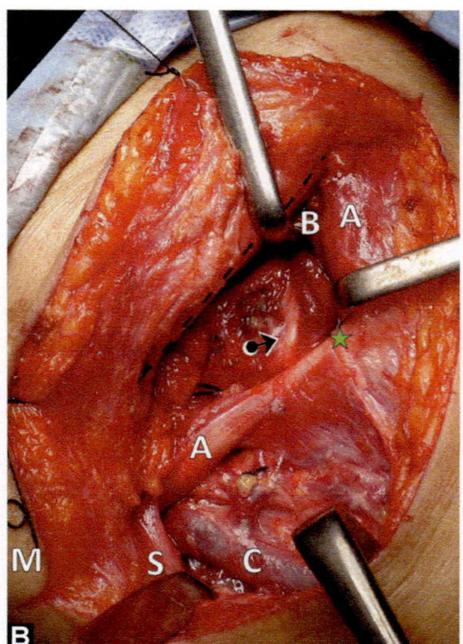

Q. 95. This image was taken during an oncologic surgery for tongue carcinoma. The submandibular gland was retracted downward on the left and the opposite view at the completion of surgery.

a. What is the likely surgery performed?

b. Identify the structures as numbered.

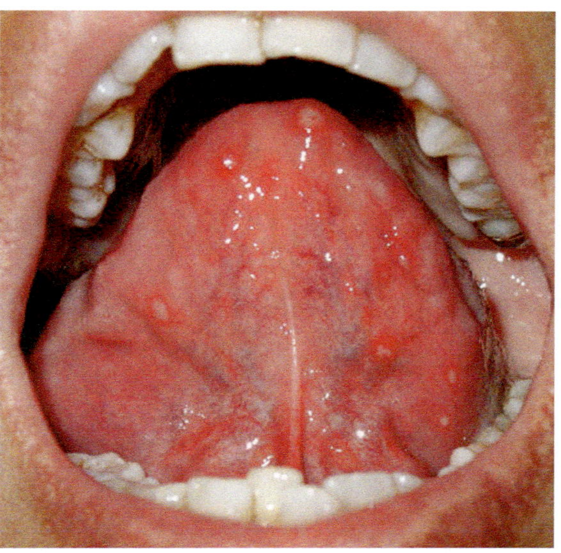

Q. 96. This gentleman presented with recurrent painful tongue lesions which usually lasted for few days.

a. Describe the lesions.
b. What is the diagnosis?
c. How would you manage this patient optimally?

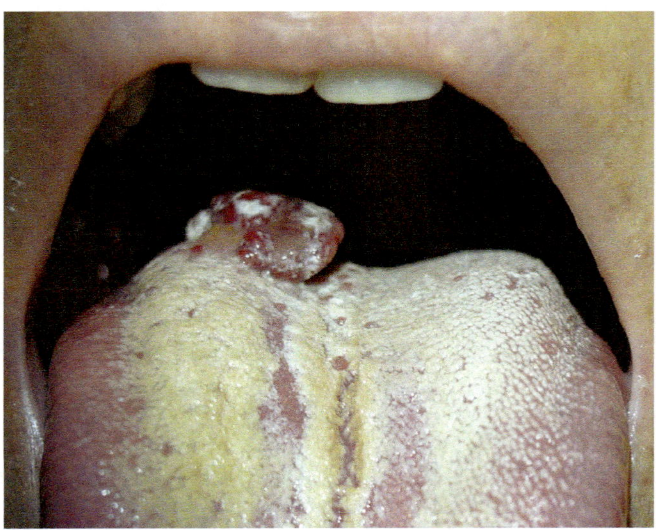

Q. 97. This is the image of the tongue of a female patient who presented with complaint of blood stained to frank bleeding from the mouth.

a. Describe the lesion shown.
b. What is the most likely diagnosis?
c. Describe the methods for its removal and justify the reasons.

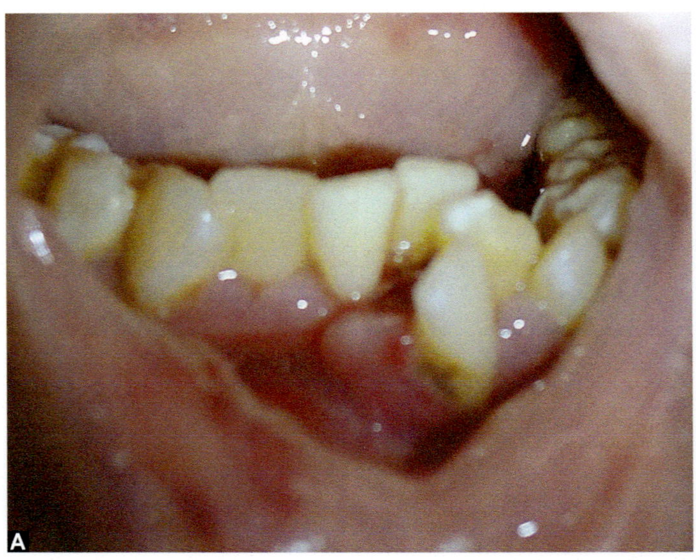

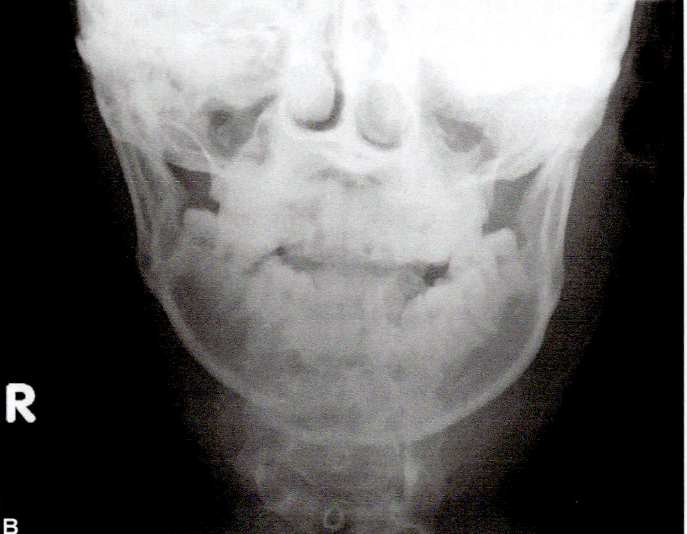

Q. 98. A 21-year-old lady was involved in a car accident and sustained multiple injuries involving the face and lower limb. Oral cavity examination was done and X-ray ordered. Her limb injuries were managed by the orthopedic team.

a. Describe the findings of both the images.
b. Give the diagnosis.
c. What other injuries should not be missed?
d. Outline further management of this patient giving focus on the facial injury.

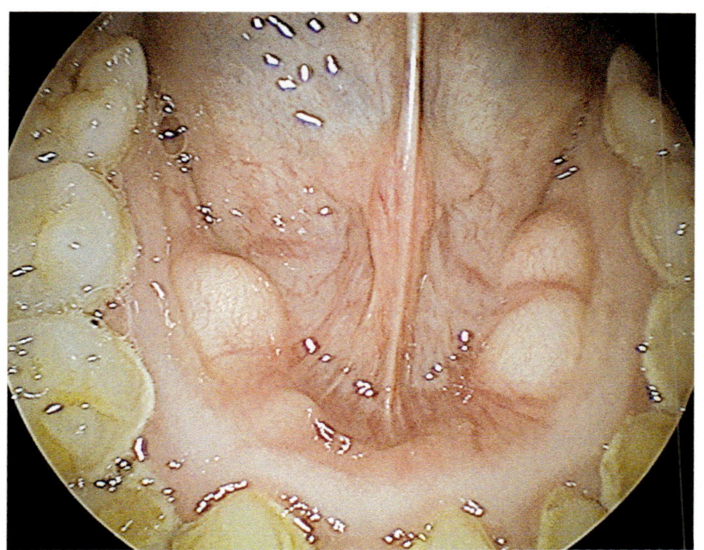

Q. 99. This is the appearance of the floor of mouth.

a. Describe the findings and give the diagnosis.

b. Should it be treated?

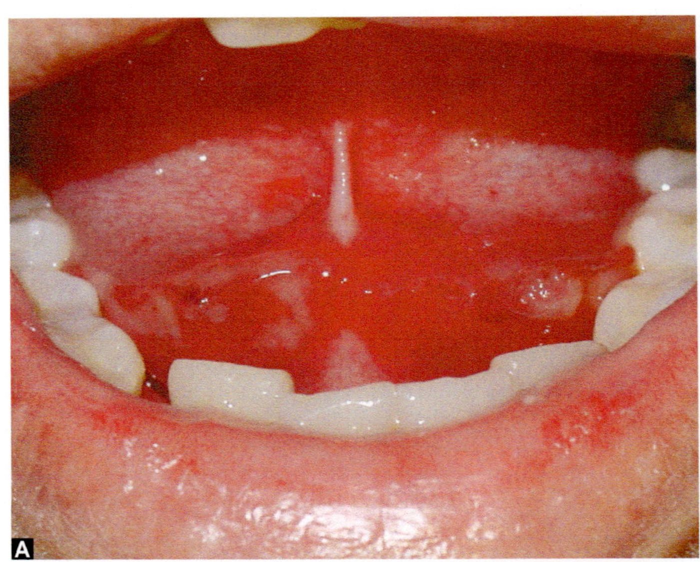

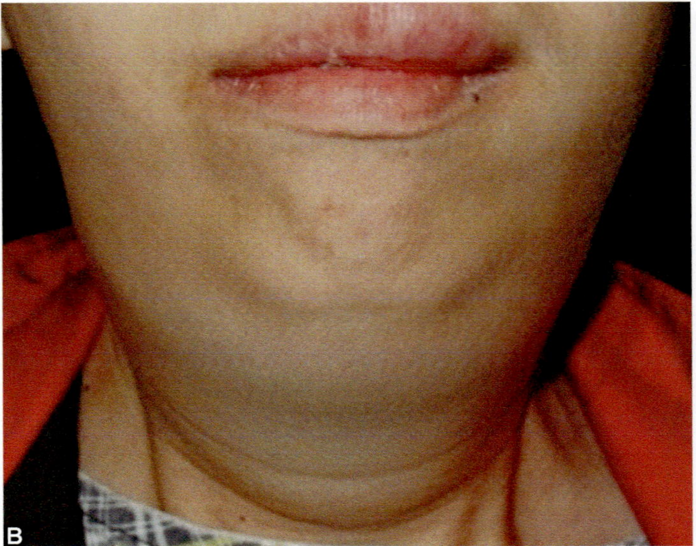

Q. 100. This lady presented with fever and swollen neck of few days durations. Blood test showed leukocytosis and culture showed no growth.

a. What is the diagnosis?
b. How is this condition managed?

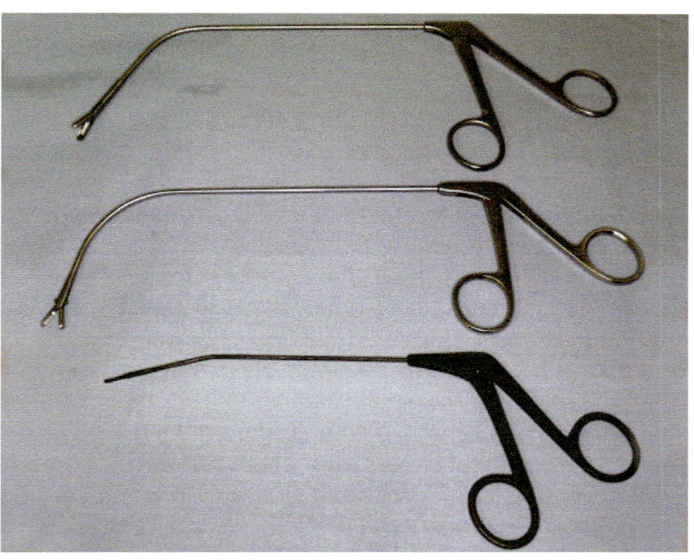

Q. 101. These instruments were designed to be used for oro-and hypopharyngeal procedures.

a. Name the instruments.

b. What are its clinical uses?

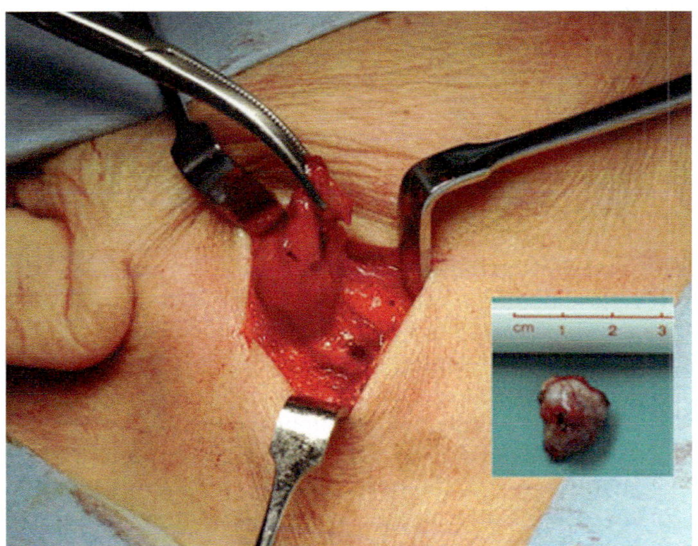

Q. 102. This female patient presented with a painless neck swelling. A diagnostic surgery under local anesthesia was performed.

a. What type of surgery is being demonstrated?

b. Give its indications.

c. Name an alternative technique and its justification.

Answers

77. a. Painless preauricular swelling includes parotid tumors and metastatic lymph nodes. The majority of these tumors are benign particularly pleomorphic adenoma and its growth is slow and gradual; thus no discernable pain will be noted as in this patient. However, the presence of pain or facial nerve palsy would favor a malignant tumor, e.g. high-grade mucoepidermoid tumor, adenoid cystic carcinoma (CA) or otherwise a malignant transformation from longstanding pleomorphic adenoma (rare).

b. Fine needle aspiration cytology (FNAC) would determine the nature of swelling, especially in differentiating, whether it is benign or malignant. Computed tomography (CT) scan will delineate the extent of involvement by tumor. Superficial parotidectomy with preservation of facial nerve (with aid of nerve monitor or stimulator) would be carried out for pleomorphic adenoma. For malignant tumor, total or extended parotidectomy with or without postoperative radiotherapy should be performed depending on its extent. Patient need to be informed of facial nerve palsy as the nerve may need to be sacrificed if involved by tumor.

78. a.
1. Facial nerve trunk
2. Temporozygomatic branch
3. Cervicofacial branch
4. Buccal branch
5. Marginal mandibular branch
6. Cervical branch
7. Posterior belly of digastric
8. Internal jugular vein
9. Sternomastoid muscle (retracted laterally)
10. Deep lobe of parotid.

Arrow points to mastoid tip area.

b. Several landmarks can be used to identify facial nerve; namely tragal pointer, mastoid process, posterior belly of digastric, and tympanomastoid suture. The nerve is 1 cm deep and inferior to tragal pointer (the tragal cartilage end); the nerve passes downward, forward and laterally, immediately above the upper border of the posterior belly of digastric, lateral and slightly posterior to the base of styloid process; the nerve bisects the angle between the two pieces of bone (the anterior border of the mastoid process and the vaginal process of tympanic bone) at the tympanomastoid suture. In difficult cases, the peripheral branch can be traced upto the main nerve trunk (retrograde approach).

79. There is bilateral tonsillar hypertrophy (Grade II-III) (Grade I no tonsillar enlargement, Grade IV kissing tonsils). The history points to chronic tonsillitis in which there is recurrent infection with normal phase in between. Treatment depends on the frequency of infection and morbidity experienced by patient. Tonsillectomy is advised when the attack is too frequent and in those requiring frequent medical leave from work or school. In addition, this would relief snoring in some patients, who have obstructive symptom related to its enlargement.

80. a. There is a thick mucopus emanating from the left tonsillar crypts with an adherent membrane of similar nature coating the right tonsil and the posterior pharyngeal wall. The tonsillar pillars and uvula were inflamed and edematous.

b. This finding is typical of acute follicular tonsillitis. However, the possibility of infectious mononucleosis should be considered based on the findings of multiple cervical lymphadenopathy.

c. Dehydration with electrolytes imbalance, septicemia, and scarlet fever. Patient with infectious mononucleosis may develop rashes upon taking ampicillin.

d. In view of poor oral intake and dehydration, this patient needs hospital admission. Intravenous fluid and antibiotic are given until the patient can tolerate better orally. Full blood count will show leukocytosis with a left shift in bacterial tonsillitis and lymphocytosis in viral tonsillitis including infectious mononucleosis.

81. a. X-ray showed a sharp radiopaque shadow in cervical esophagus opposite C6/C7 cervical vertebrae. There is no air column or significant prevertebral soft tissue swelling, which will also indicate the presence of foreign body. This would be most likely due to foreign body impaction particularly fishbone, which is a common dish served in Southeast Asian countries.

b. The patient needs an esophagoscopy examination under anesthesia to remove the foreign body. If the patient is unfit to undergo general anesthesia (GA), removal can also be done under sedation in endoscopy suite using flexible esophagoscopy. Nasogastric tube should be inserted if the mucosa lacerated and postoperatively the patient monitored for signs of complications like fever, tachycardia, and central chest pain.

82. The swelling appears to be located at the carotid triangle of the neck and anterior to sternomastoid muscle at its junction of upper one-third and lower two-third. The cause of swelling here would include cervical lymph node, non-Hodgkin lymphoma, branchial cyst, and carotid body tumor. Considering the patient's age and clinical presentation, branchial cyst would be the most likely diagnosis. It appears as a well-defined cystic lesion anteromedial to the sternomastoid muscle. It is the most common type of branchial arch anomaly and usually present in young age patient. Computed tomography scan revealed a homodense well-defined rounded lesion. Treatment is by the complete excision of the cyst.

83. a. The barium swallow revealed a persistent anterior narrowing defect opposite the level of C5/C6 vertebrae.

b. This is most likely due to an esophageal web. The clinical feature of dysphagia and investigation results revealed hypochromic microcytic anemia, which is typical in this condition.

c. There is a small risk of malignancy associated with the web. Thus, a thorough esophageal examination should be carried out. Usually, the esophageal web appears as a crescentic narrowing just at/below the cricopharyngeal sphincter. Therefore, attention must be paid at this area and examination should be proceeded slowly. Biopsy should be taken and followed by dilatation procedures. Iron deficiency anemia need to be corrected and dietary advice given. This condition is also known as Paterson-Kelly and Plummer-Vinson syndrome.

84. These are esophageal bougies used for dilating strictures. Usually, the smallest size that fits into the narrowing be used first followed by subsequent sizes, until adequate dilatation achieved. Dilatation should be stopped if there is bleeding as this would indicate a significant injury to submucosal layer that would predispose to further fibrosis and that will worsen the stricture. The bougies may need to be chilled first to stiffen its tip for the ease of insertion. In addition, this would also help to reduce postprocedural mucosal hyperemia and edema. Care is taken not to overdilate in a single session as to reduce the risk of tear or perforation. Repeated procedure may need to be done depending on the patient's relief of symptom.

85. a. These pictures are characteristic of rheumatoid arthritis. They have joint pain and demonstrate the classical finger deformities as shown in the picture.

b. Patients usually present to ENT clinic with dryness of mouth and eyes, and neck swellings are typically grouped under secondary Sjogren's syndrome.

c. The picture of lip indicates a sublabial biopsy that is usually performed to confirm the diagnosis of Sjogren's syndrome, where typical lymphocyte infiltration is seen.

86. a. The provisional diagnosis would be a branchial fistula/sinus. This characteristically opens at the inferior part of the neck just anterior to sternocleidomastoid muscle. It is due to an embryological anomaly due to incomplete fusion of branchial cleft. Patients usually present with recurrent discharge from the fistula/sinus. This track usually extends upward between the bifurcations of the carotid arteries and subsequently ends in either the lower part of tonsil or pyriform fossa depending on which branchial cleft is involved. Management is via surgical excision where the entire tract is removed totally.

b. Similar fistulas can occur according to the branchial cleft/arch involved. First arch fistulas can open into bony-cartilaginous junction part of ear canal while the second arch fistula can open in upper neck and traverses through the parotid and facial nerve.

87. a. The cumulated secretion revealed dual layered color with the lower one hemoserous and the upper milky white. This is typically seen in chylous leak in which the thoracic duct has been severed as it entered the brachiocephalic vein in the lower part of neck on the left side. As homeostasis secured in the next few days the content of the bottle would be completely creamy white in color.

b. This complication can be managed conservatively initially by giving nothing by mouth but putting the patient on intravenous fluid (Note: fatty food will make it worse). However, this would be insufficient for the patient postoperatively (catabolic state and tissue healing phase); thus total parenteral nutrition will be usually necessary. Immediate exploration is rarely needed, as in majority of the cases it will be resolved spontaneously, unless it is a high output leak. Care must be taken during neck dissection on the left side and the presence of clear fluid near the lower anterior neck would indicate severed thoracic duct that should be repaired immediately. In some cases of persistent leak, radiotherapy can be started early and this will seal the leak.

88. a. A bifid uvula.

b. The possibility of submucous cleft palate should be considered. Thus, the palate needs to be palpated carefully to look for the defect. This condition may predispose to Eustachian tube dysfunction and glue ear, especially in children. Adenoid removal is to be avoided as it may worsen the ear problem. In this patient, no submucous cleft was found and the ear showed mild retraction bilaterally without evidence of effusion.

c. Audiometry and tympanometry need to be done to assess the hearing loss and tympanic membrane compliance. Valsalva maneuver is to be advised, and Myringstomy and grommet insertion can be considered if the hearing loss is significant.

89. There appears to be a swelling attached to three distinct cord-like branches, most probably facial nerve as this is a parotid surgery. The swelling is most likely to be a facial nerve schwannoma, which is a benign tumor of the facial nerve. This can be found in other nerves in the body and can be malignant in some cases. These patients usually do not have a facial nerve palsy during early stages and present with a parotid swelling. Fine needle aspiration cytology is useful but is not foolproof. It is often only discovered during surgery and thus it is needed to inform every parotid surgery patient of the small but real chance of facial nerve schwannoma. The management consist of excision of the tumor with adequate margin (confirmed with frozen section) and as far as possible, nerve grafting (sural or greater auricular according to surgeon's preference) in the same sitting. Recovery is quite good but the patient must be warned that recovery can take months (6 months and more) and the facial nerve function will never be back to normal; usually House-Brackmann Grade III–IV. Recurrence of tumor is possible and thus a negative frozen section of the margin is important.

90. a. This appears to be neurofibromatosis or von Recklinghausen's disease. This is an autosomal dominant hereditary disorder, in which patients have multiple neuromas that can present anywhere in the body. In rare instances, it can be due to spontaneous mutation. Other features of this condition include café-au-lait spots and plexiform fibroma.

b. Clinical presentation depends on the site of the neuroma. In this patient, the neck swelling is probably due to a neuroma in the parapharyngeal space. Involvement of cranial nerves or in the spine can result in fatal outcome. Bilateral vestibular schwannomas are atypical presentation, where patients present with hearing loss and imbalance due to brainstem compression. Management consists of excision of tumors that are symptomatic.

91. a. This patient had a radial forearm free flap (Chinese free flap) that is usually used to reconstruct defects in head and neck areas in ENT specialty.

b. Considering the lateral tongue as the area of primary excision, this would most probably be due to the tongue CA usually squamous cell. As the area of excision in the tongue appears to be less than half, then it is very likely to be a partial glossectomy. The degree of tongue excision depends on the size of the primary lesion with a good tumor-free surgical margin. Thus, it can be a hemiglossectomy (half of tongue), subtotal or total glossectomy depending on the size of primary lesion. Neck dissection is also carried out in cases of clinically or/and radiologically proven neck metastases.

c. Early cases without neck node metastasis can be treated with radiotherapy.

92. This is a picture that shows the elevation of a deltopectoral flap. It is a pedicled flap that is based on the upper four perforators of the internal thoracic artery and used quite frequently in reconstruction of defects in head and neck oncologic surgery, especially in oral cavity, cheek and floor of mouth. The main disadvantage is that it entails a two-stage procedure that requires a staged release of the flap upon the take up of the recipient site after several weeks.

93. a. This photo shows an intraoperative view of removal of a midline anterior neck cyst below the hyoid bone.

b. This appears to be a thyroglossal cyst based on the location of the lesion.

c. This operation is called Sistrunk's operation. A transverse midline skin incision is made over the swelling and subplatysmal flap is raised. The lesion is mobilized from the surrounding structures until its neck is identified, which usually runs through the hyoid bone. The hyoid body is then excised and the tract is followed usually until it ends at the base of tongue.

94. a. The lateral neck X-ray reveals widening of retropharyngeal space and the CT scan reveals a hypodense lesion at the retropharyngeal space.

b. This appears to be a retropharyngeal abscess.

c. She needs to be admitted for hydration, to control her blood glucose with insulin sliding scale, intravenous antibiotics and incision and drainage of the abscess under GA.

95. a. This appears to be a selective neck dissection most probably a supraomohyoid neck dissection with wide excision of tongue CA.

b. A: Digastric muscle

B: Mylohyoid muscle

C: Internal jugular vein

S: Sternomastoid muscle

M: Mastoid tip area

SM: Submandibular gland

Star: Digastric tendon

Black arrow: Hypoglossal nerve

White arrow: Lingual nerve.

96. a. There are multiple ulcers noted at ventral surface of the tongue as well as the floor of the mouth.

b. The diagnosis is aphthous ulcers of the oral cavity.

c. She needs oral gargle with lignocaine and triamcinolone gel (e.g. oral aid) to reduce the pain and promote the healing process.

97. a. The image shows a bluish-red fungating swelling arising from right paramedian aspect of the distal anterior two-third of the tongue.

b. The most likely diagnosis is tongue hemangioma.

c. The mass should be removed using coagulation diathermy to coagulate its base and then removed in the same setting. This would reduce intraoperative bleeding. Alternatively, bipolar radiosurgical device can be used such as Surgitron with the parameter set at cut and coagulation mode.

98. a. The images showed discontinuity of the lower teeth and the alveolus with minor bruise of inner aspect of the lower lip.

b. The most likely diagnosis is close fracture of the mandible (parasymphysis).

c. Other injuries should not be missed are temporomandibular joint injuries, e.g. effusion or dislocation, other craniofacial injuries, intracranial injuries and neck injury especially involving the airway.

d. Further management of this patient focusing on the mandibular injury is open reduction with wire fixation of the fractured segment.

Analgesics and anti-inflammatory medication need to be given adequately.

99. a. The image shows multiple rounded lesions arising from the inner aspect of the mandible. The gingiva and teeth are normal. The diagnosis is torus mandibularis which is a slow-growing benign bony mass.

b. This lesions can be left alone as it is usually asymptomatic and found by chance.

100. a. The most likely diagnosis is Ludwig's angina.

b. She should be admitted and started on parenteral antibiotics. Beware of the upper airway obstruction as the submental swelling will push the tongue backward and obstruct the upper airway. Intubation or tracheostomy can be performed to relieve the upper airway obstruction. Incision and drainage can be performed if abscess is formed. A transverse incision extending from one angle of mandible to the other is made with vertical opening of the midline musculature of tongue by using a blunt hemostat.

101. a. These are angled biopsy forceps (the upper two instruments) with an upturn and sideway biting angles used typically for hypopharyngeal area. The lower black-colored instrument is Kaluskar forceps which is widely used for the removal of foreign body at tongue base area.

b. These instruments are used clinically for removal of foreign body and taking biopsy.

102. a. The surgery being performed is excisional lymph node biopsy.

b. It is indicated to confirm the diagnosis by histopathological examination usually necessary in suspected lymphoma.

c. The alternative technique is FNAC as this can be performed as office clinic procedure with 80–90% sensitivity (operator dependent).

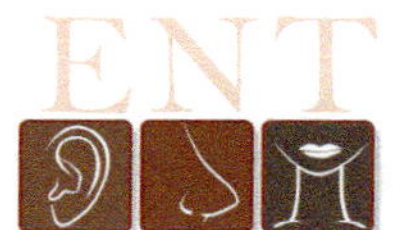

4 LARYNGOLOGY

Questions

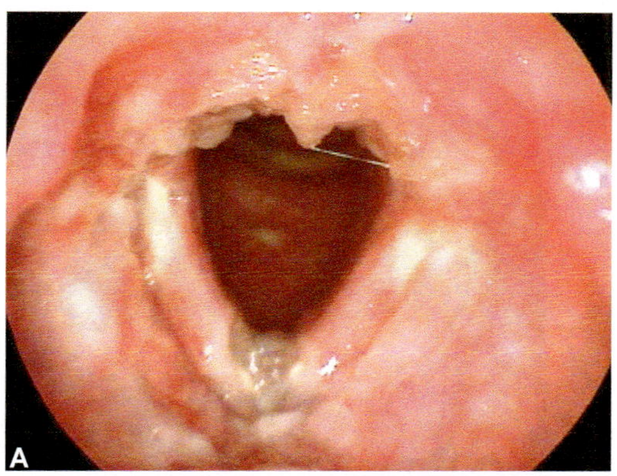

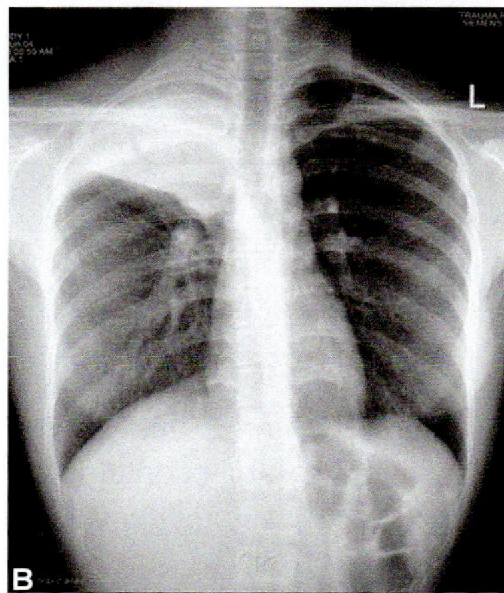

Q. 103. An immigrant lady presented with the history of hoarseness preceded by chronic cough. Laryngeal examination was performed and a chest X-ray ordered. Mantoux test was negative.

a. Describe the laryngeal lesion as shown.
b. Describe the chest X-ray findings.
c. What is the most likely diagnosis?
d. How would this patient be managed further?

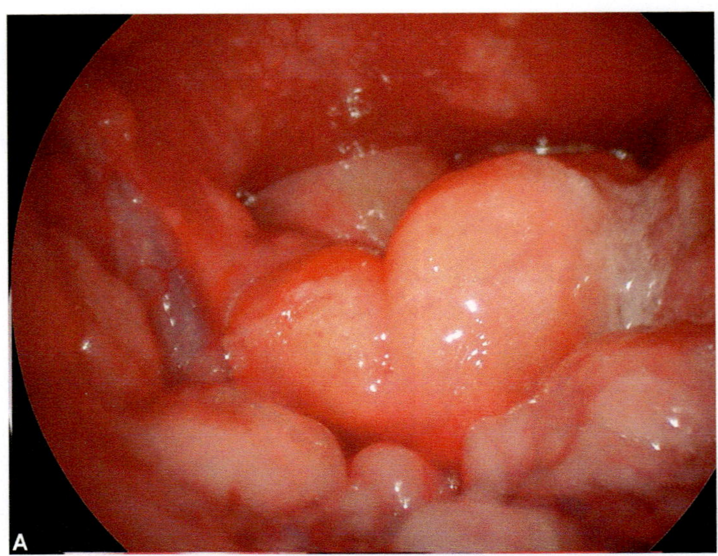

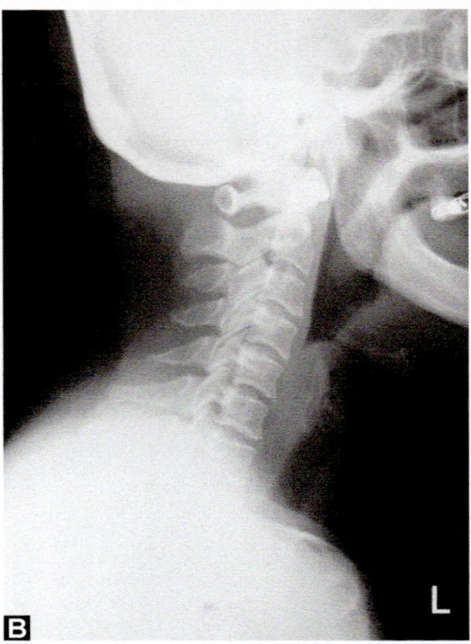

Q. 104. A young Malay lady presented with sudden onset of hoarseness and stridor after ingesting tablet containing evening primrose oil. Laryngeal endoscopic view and lateral soft tissue X-ray attached.

a. Describe the X-ray findings.
b. Explain the endoscopic findings.
c. What is the likely diagnosis?
d. How would this patient be managed further?

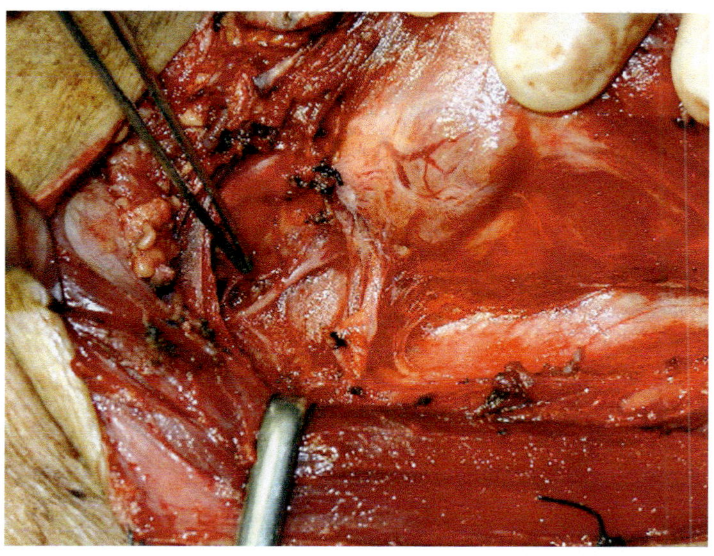

Q. 105. This is an intraoperative view of a patient, who is undergoing a total thyroidectomy.

a. Describe what is being highlighted.
b. What would happen if this is severed or damaged and how to avoid this injury?

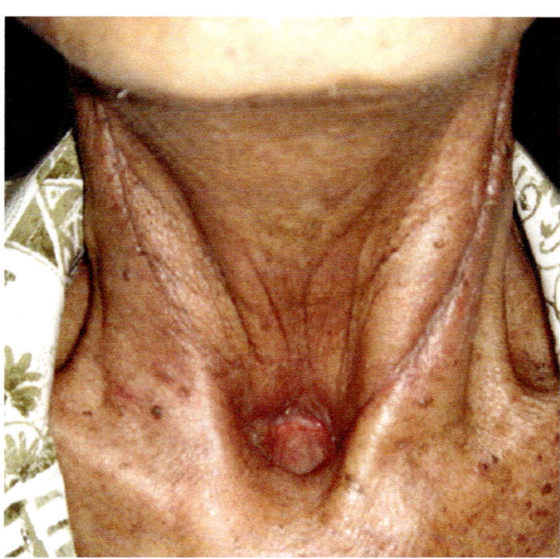

Q. 106. This is the neck image of a patient, who had his larynx removed for the recurrence carcinoma of larynx.

a. Describe the findings.
b. What is needed to be considered for this patient?

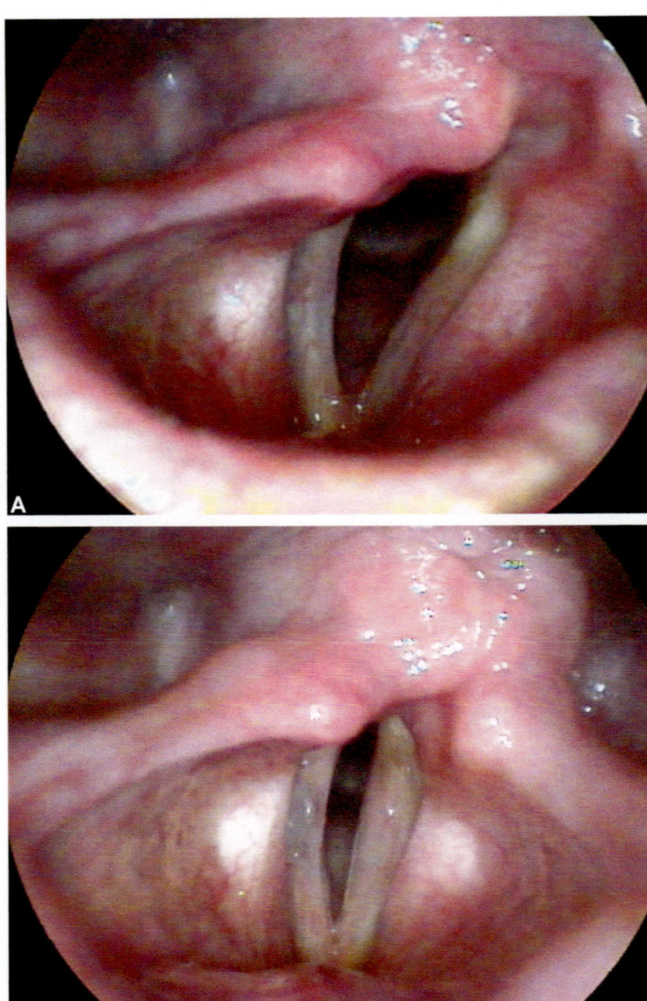

Q. 107. This patient presented with a chronic breathy voice after thyroid surgery performed many years earlier. Videostroboscopy was performed and still images taken during phonation are enclosed.

a. Describe the findings and likely diagnosis.
b. How would this patient be managed further?

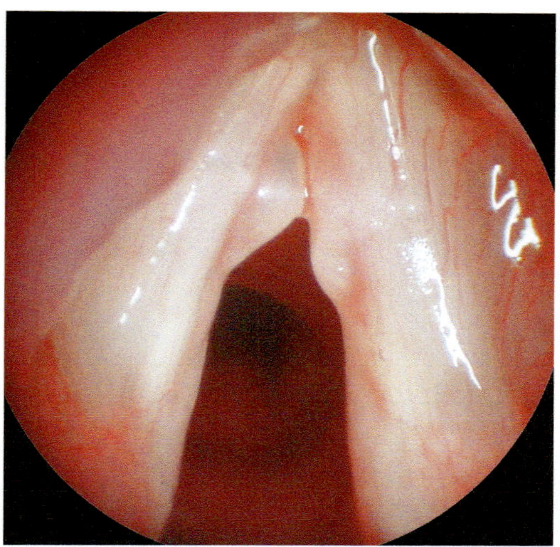

Q. 108. A 9-year-old school boy presented with history of hoarse voice for 3 years duration.

Examination under anesthesia was performed and findings were as shown.

a. Describe the findings.
b. What is the likely diagnosis?
c. What is the subsequent treatment?

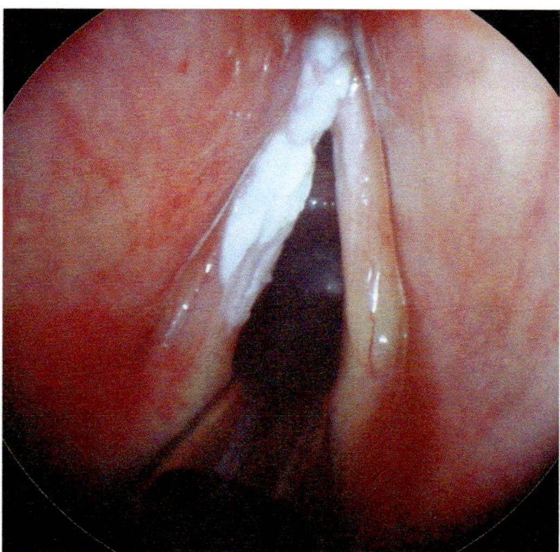

Q. 109. This patient presented with the hoarseness of voice for few months duration. He gave the history of chronic smoking earlier, but no alcohol consumption noted. Direct laryngoscopy was performed and intraoperative image was as shown.

a. Describe the findings.
b. What is the likely diagnosis?
c. How would this patient be managed further?

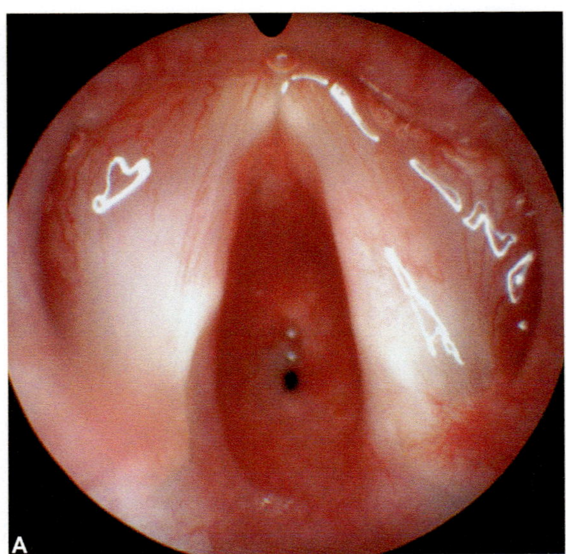

A

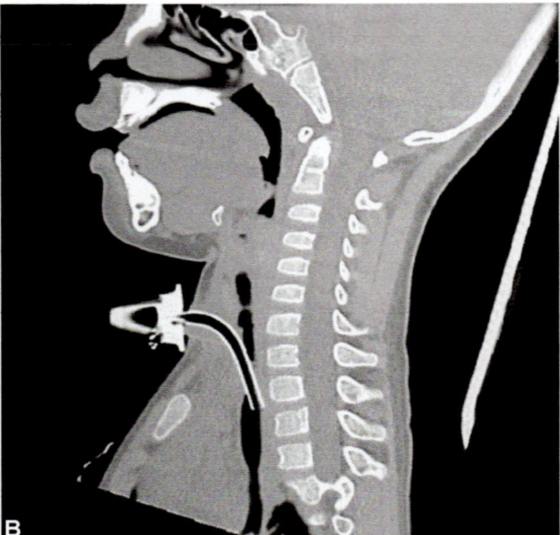

B

Q. 110. A 1-year-old child presented with worsening stridor and difficulty in breathing for which emergency tracheostomy was performed. Computed tomography scan was ordered and subsequently the child scheduled for direct laryngoscopy. He was born prematurely at 34 weeks and managed in pediatric intensive care unit, after which he was discharged well.

a. Describe the findings on direct laryngoscopy and the Computed tomography scan findings.
b. What is the diagnosis?
c. How would this child be managed further?

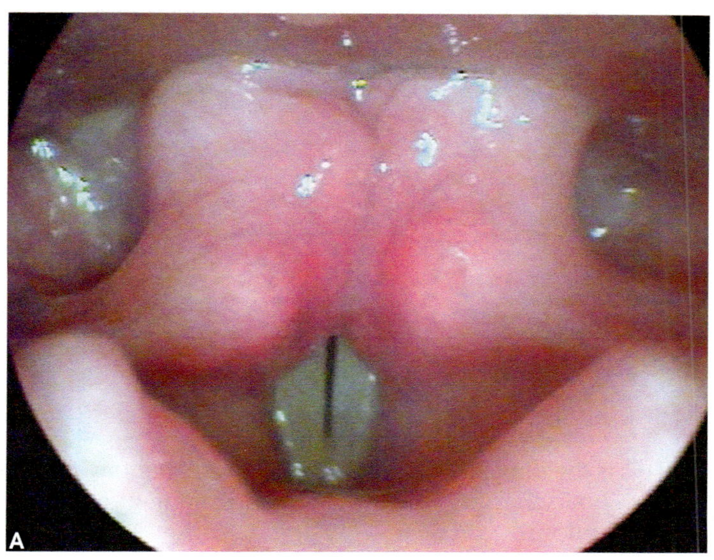

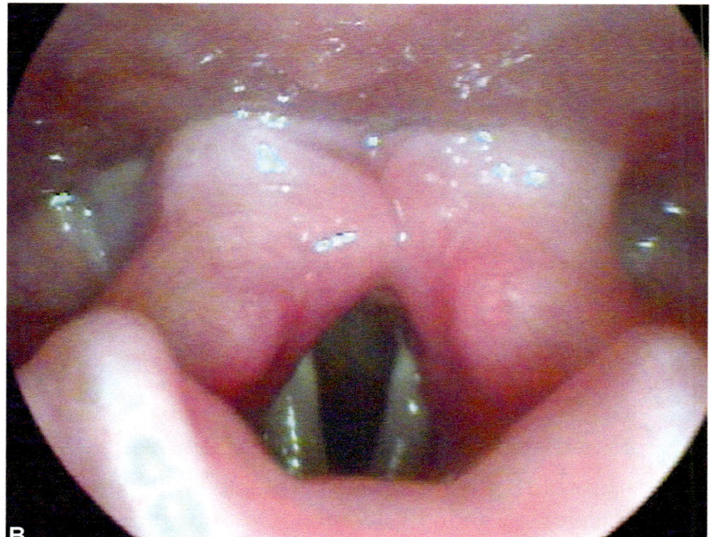

Q. 111. This young patient presented to outpatient ENT clinic with a feeling of food sticking in the throat and fluctuating voice change usually worse in the morning. There were no nasal symptoms or recent respiratory tract infection. Videostroboscopy was performed and still images on adduction and abduction were shown, respectively.

a. Describe the findings.
b. What is the most likely diagnosis?
c. How would this case proceed?

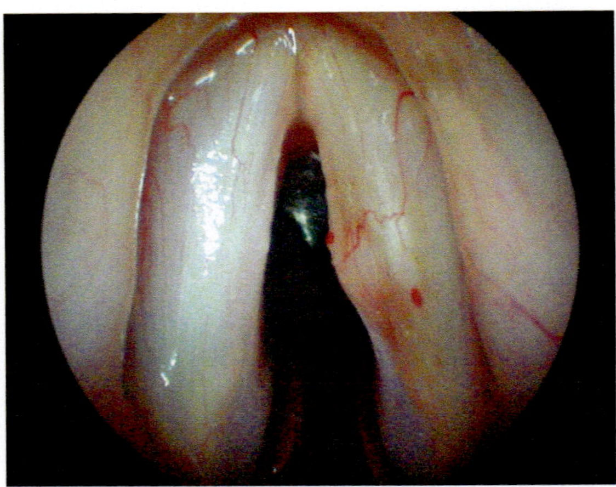

Q. 112. This is the direct laryngoscopic view of a patient, who presented with hoarseness of voice. Describe the findings and its clinical implications.

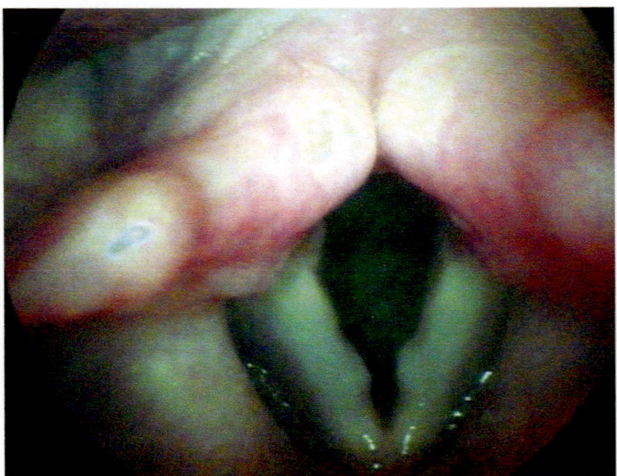

Q. 113. A 9-year-old prefect schoolboy presented with persistent change of voice over 6 months duration. On duty, he gave instructions and sometimes needed to talk louder than usual.

a. Describe the findings.
b. Give the diagnosis.
c. How would this boy be managed optimally?
d. What is the role of surgery in this case?

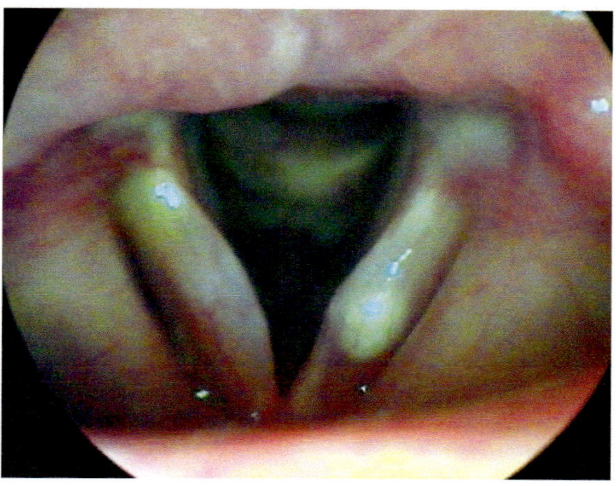

Q. 114. A schoolteacher presented with hoarse voice for 8 months duration, when she posed difficulty in teaching. She never had similar complaints before. On consultation her voice was raspy, and endoscopic evaluation showed no evidence of vocal fold palsy. Still image was as shown.

a. Describe the findings.
b. What is the diagnosis?
c. Is there any role of speech therapy in this case?
d. How would this lesion be treated?

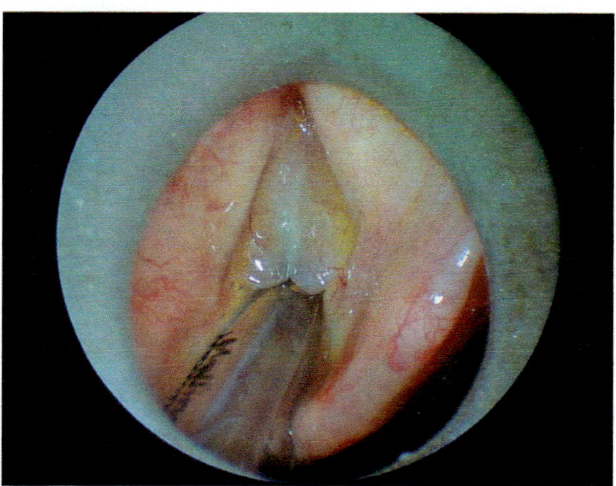

Q. 115. A chronic smoker presented with severe hoarseness for about an year duration. On consultation, his voice was grave in nature and has limited projection. Endoscopic assessment and microlaryngeal surgery was performed.

a. Describe the intraoperative findings.
b. What is the diagnosis?
c. Describe the definitive procedure that needs to be performed.
d. How would this patient be advised postoperatively with regards to the prognosis?

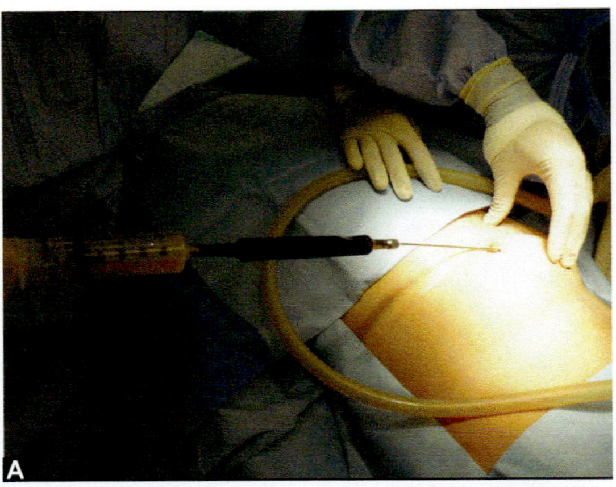

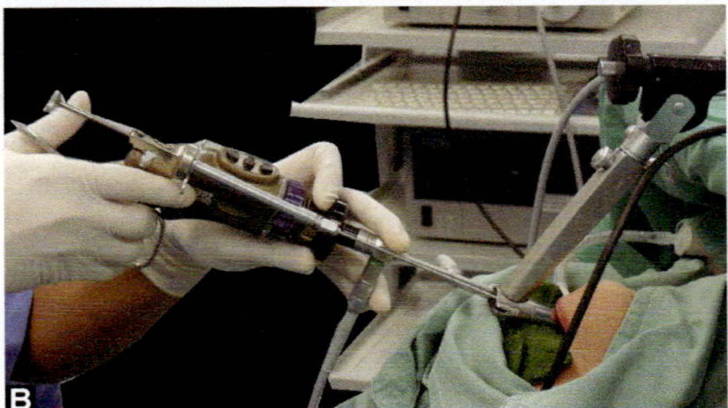

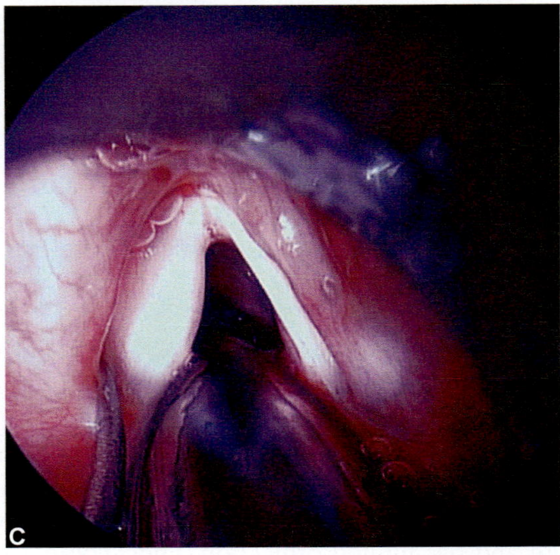

Q. 116. These images showed surgery being performed for voice improvement in adductor vocal fold palsy.

a. What thyroplasty technique is being shown?
b. List the advantage of this surgery as compared to others.
c. What potential complications can occur?
d. Name the injection instrument being used.

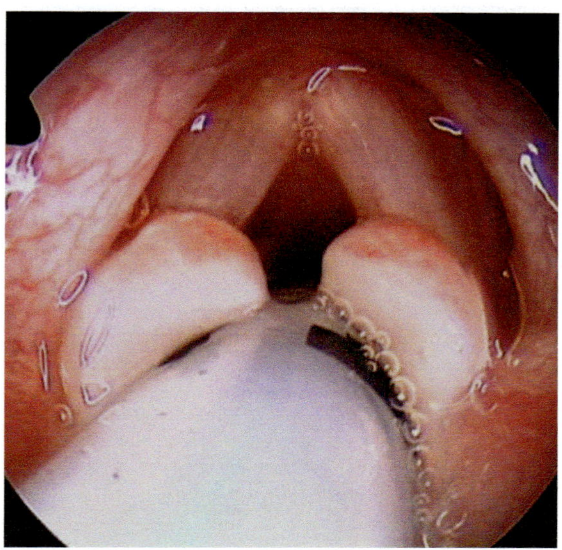

Q. 117. A child was intubated due to upper airway obstruction for 10 days duration. Intraoperative laryngeal assessment was performed prior to definitive surgical intervention.

a. Describe the findings.
b. What is the diagnosis?
c. List the sequelae if this lesion is not being managed optimally.

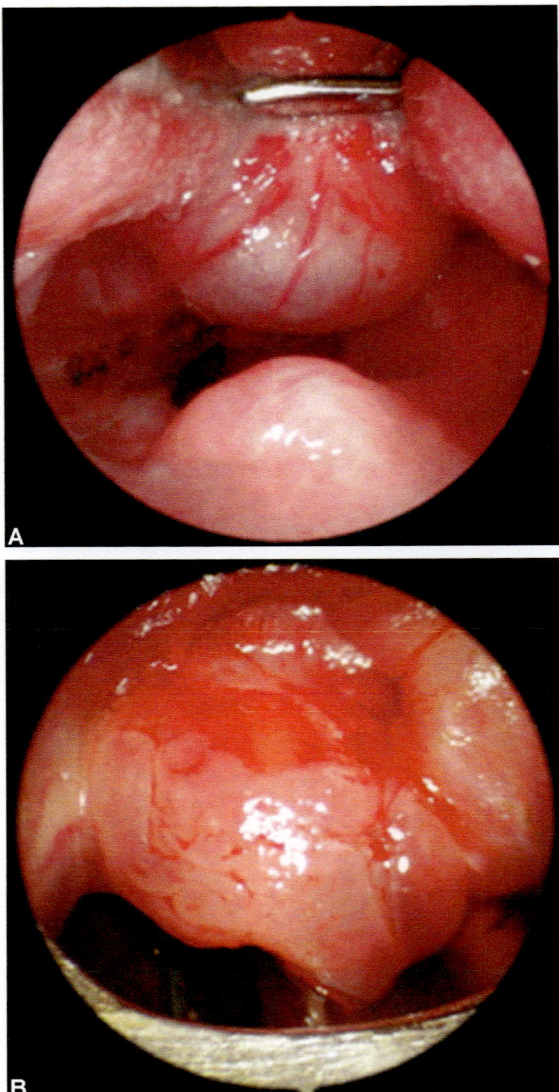

Q. 118. This is an intraoperative image of a 3-week-old infant, who presented with stridor. Figures shown were the pre- and postoperative views, respectively.

a. Describe the findings.
b. Give the diagnosis.
c. What surgery likely was performed?

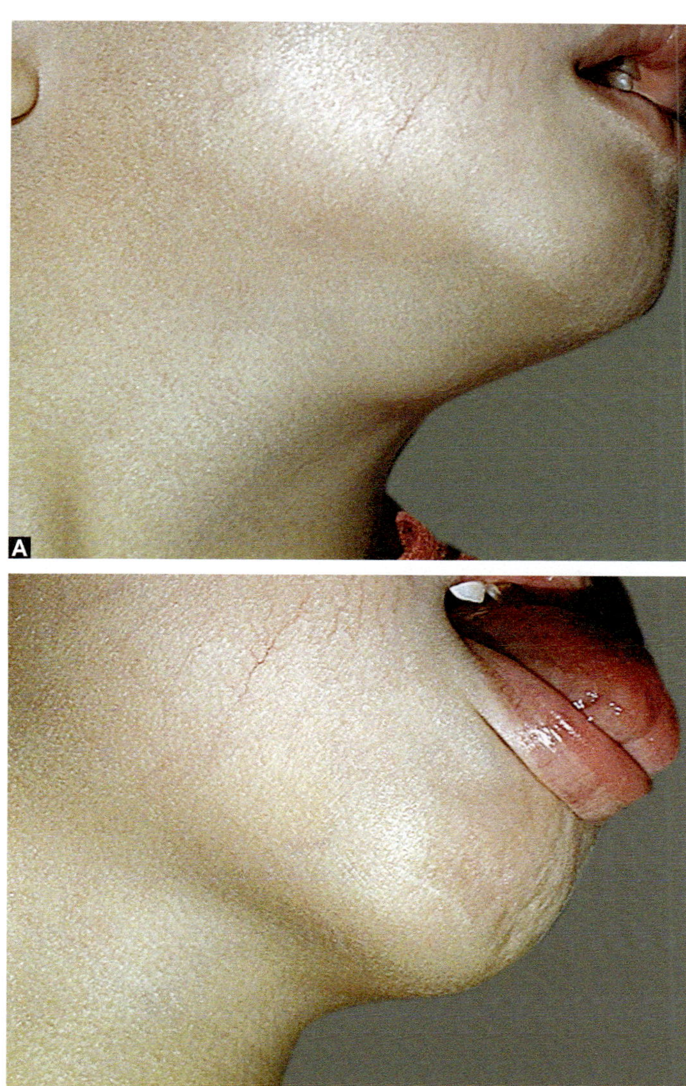

Q. 119. a. Describe the findings of these images.
b. Give the diagnosis.
c. How would this patient be managed further?

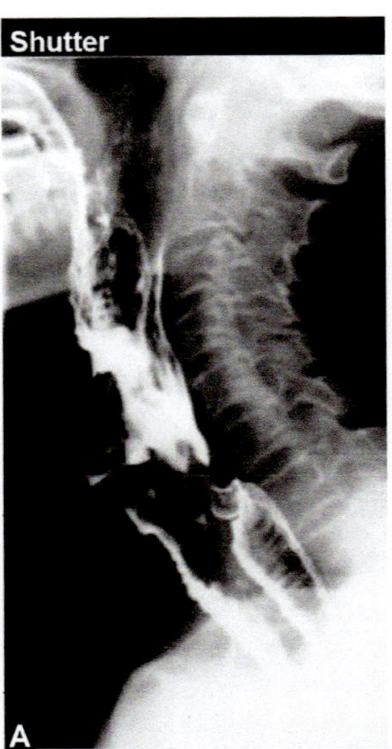

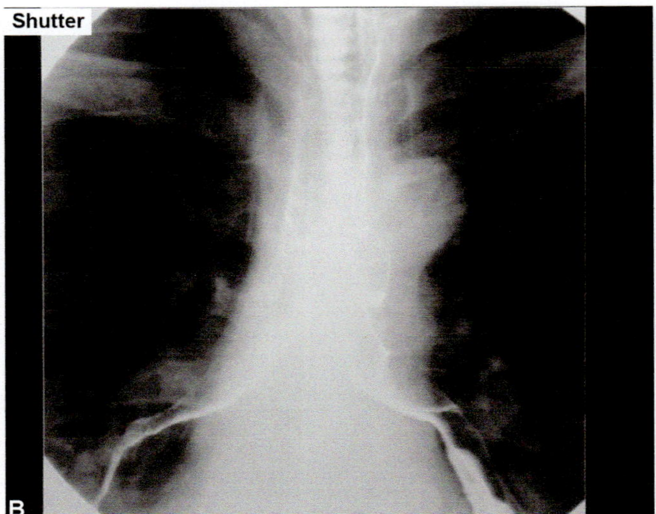

Q. 120. An elderly patient presented with progressive dysphagia to both solid and liquid. A radiological investigation was performed but he developed procedural complication.

a. Describe the findings of the radiological images.
b. What is the diagnosis?
c. Outline the management.

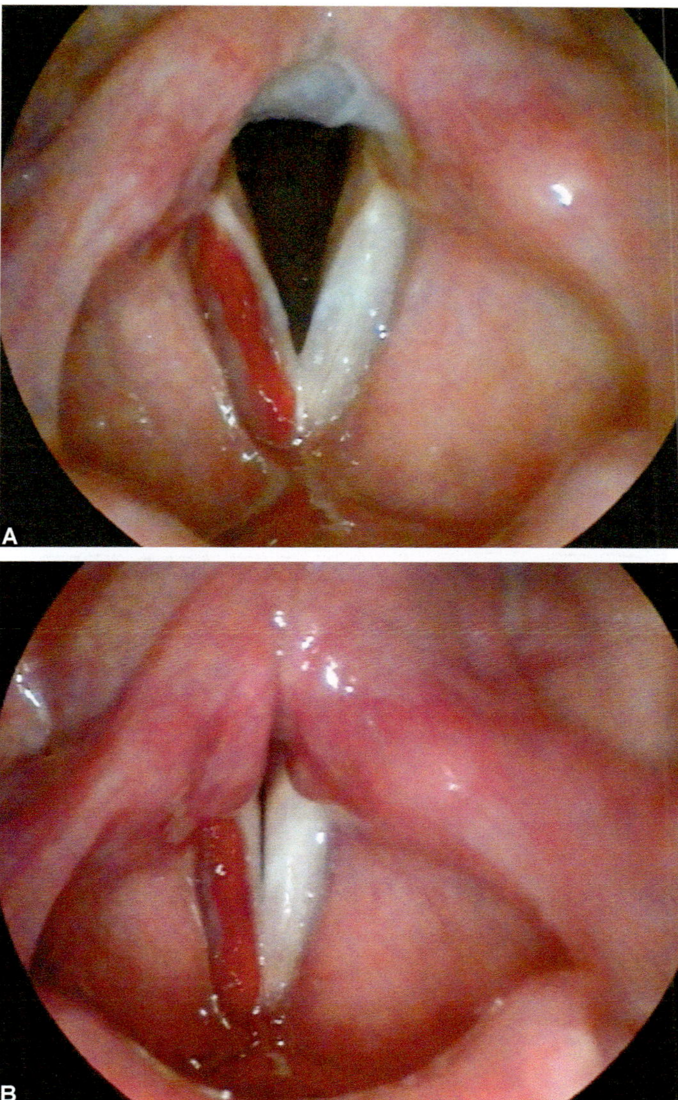

Q. 121. A 30-year-singer suddenly noted sudden change of voice and laryngeal irritation while singing. She stopped immediately and gave rest to her voice. However, her voice did not improve; she decided to get medical advice a day later.

a. Describe the laryngeal findings and give the diagnosis.
b. How is this condition treated?

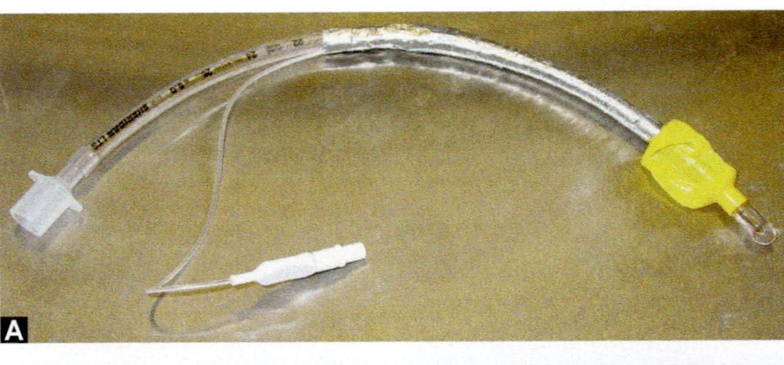

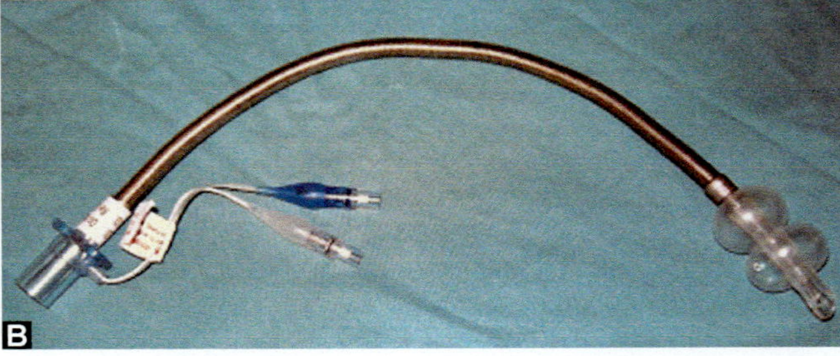

Q. 122. Compare these two endotracheal tubes and list its differences. What are the indications for its usage?

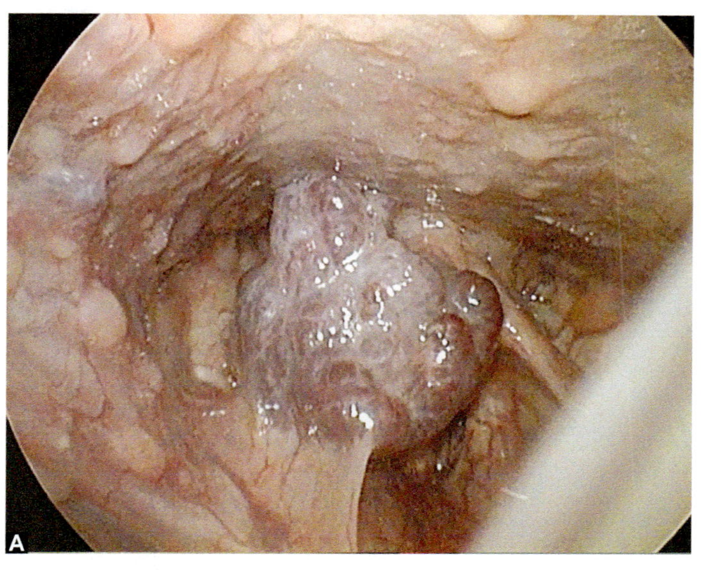

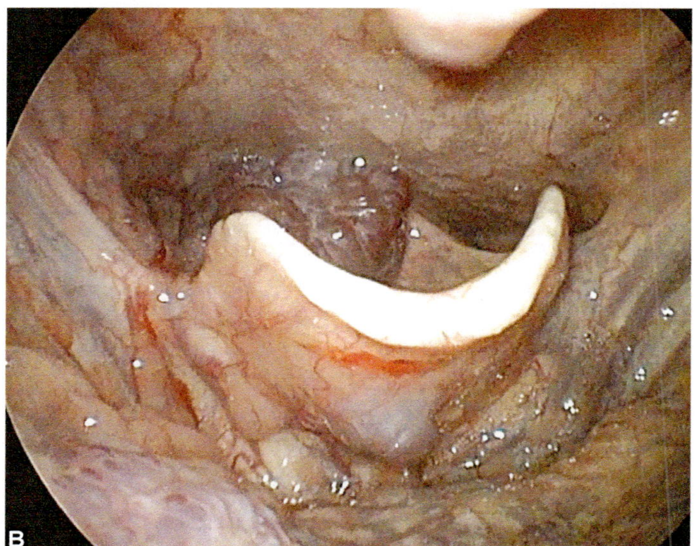

Q. 123. a. Describe the findings of these images and give possible diagnoses.
b. What further investigations should be considered?
c. How would this patient be treated?

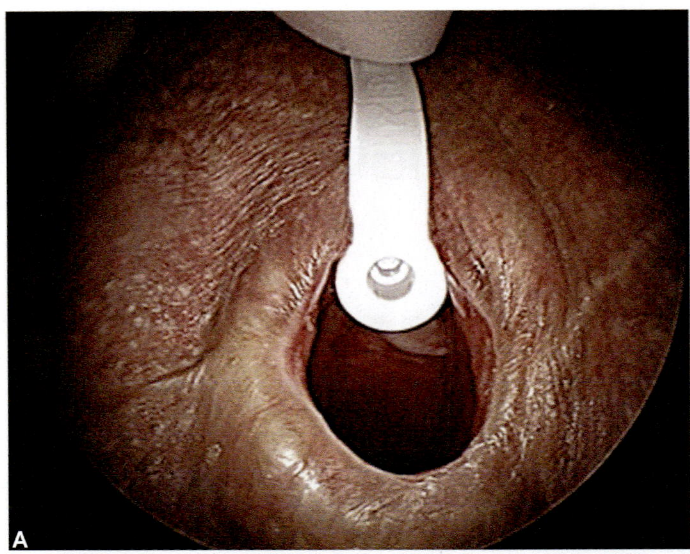

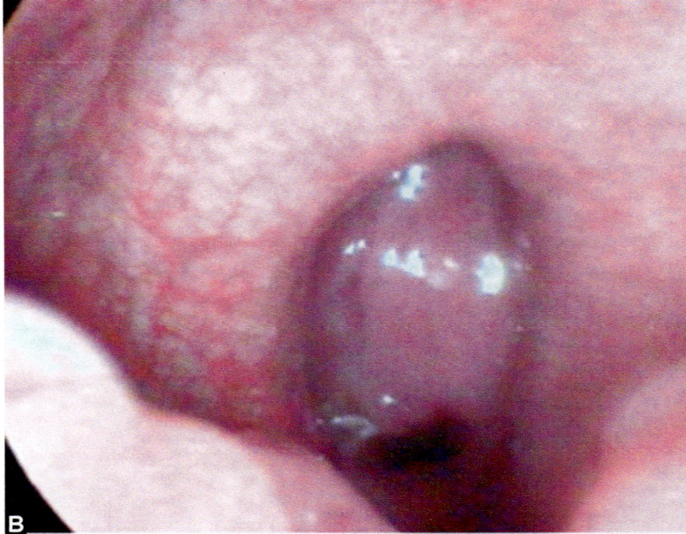

Q. 124. a. Describe the findings of these images in a patient who had total laryngectomy performed.
b. What are the advantages and disadvantages of this procedure?

Answers

103. a. Laryngeal image showed scattered grayish-white exudates, ulcerations of the vocal cords near the anterior commissure, and thickened polypoidal interarytenoid mucosa.

b. The X-ray revealed a typical wedge-shaped opacity affecting the right upper lobe and apical region, with the trachea remaining the central. This is typical in bronchopneumonia.

c. Tuberculous (TB) laryngitis is secondary to TB bronchopneumonia. History of chronic cough, which complicates into hoarseness should raise a high index of suspicion of TB. Further detailed history like fever, night sweats, loss of weight, and loss of appetite, as well as possibility of contact with patient suffering from TB must be obtained. Otherwise, immunosuppressed states need to be ruled out.

d. Full blood count (FBC), erythrocyte sedimentation rate (ESR), morning sputum for swab and cultures (x3) and Mantoux test. In this patient the FBC revealed a highly elevated ESR, positive sputum for acid-fast bacilli, but negative Mantoux test. Thus, this patient is highly infectious in an apparently non-reacting Mantoux called anergy state. Cough etiquette and wearing of suitable face mask must be followed until sputum culture becomes negative on treatment. Treatment entails combination of TB drug therapy for a period of at least 6 months. Contact tracings need to be done by local health authority and treated accordingly.

104. a. There is a thumb-shaped soft tissue swelling in the area of supraglottic larynx originating from the arytenoid area. The epiglottis is also swollen as suggested by the thickened opaque shadow just behind the base of tongue. The air bronchogram does not show any evidence of subglottic or tracheal narrowing.

b. The endoscopy view showed a markedly swollen epiglottis and edematous arytenoid mucosa with no obvious erythema or exudates seen. Pooling of saliva is not seen here.

c. Stridor in this patient occurred at supraglottic level. There is no fever, significant pain, or purulent exudates to suggest infection. In view of unfamiliar food eaten before and subsequent development of symptoms, this would be very likely due to localized hypersensitivity reaction, e.g. angioneurotic edema. Supraglottic larynx has a rich lymphatic supply and vulnerable to angioneurotic edema with fast onset of airway obstruction. If the lesion occurs repeatedly, possibility of C1 esterase deficiency needs to be considered.

d. Intravenous steroid, e.g. dexamethasone or methylprednisolone, and antihistamine would be the first-line of treatment. Endotracheal intubation is justified, in view of worsening airway caliber, while waiting for the reactions to subside. Antibiotic is not necessary.

105. a. The thyroid lobe is being retracted to the opposite side. The forceps point to the left recurrent laryngeal nerve as it ascends through the tracheoesophageal groove heading to the larynx by running behind the cricothyroid joint.

b. Ipsilateral vocal cord paresis or palsy can occur if this nerve is inadvertently severed or cut. Even excessive traction or manipulation may result in temporary loss of function called neuropraxia. The nerve need to be identified early and preserved in benign thyroid surgery. A bilateral recurrent nerve injury can occur in total thyroidectomy. Patient may present with a stridor and a normal voice. Use of nerve monitor may need to be considered in some instances, e.g. massive goiter, or in revision thyroidectomy.

106. a. Image shows surgical scars running bilaterally downward across the sternomastoid and meets at the suprasternal notch area (Gluck-Sorenson). There is an end tracheostomy in which the upper end of trachea (after the larynx resected and removed) was anastomosed directly to the skin for the purpose of breathing.

b. Firstly, the stoma need to be covered as contaminants and foreign body may enter the larynx causing bronchial irritations or pulmonary complications. Simple handkerchief or scarf can be used; otherwise commercialized bip or even stoma protector with filter can be worn. Care is taken while taking shower and of course patient can get drowned by swimming. Secondly, since the larynx was removed some form of speech rehabilitation need to be considered to enable communication. This has to be informed early to the patient and appropriate counseling and available options informed by speech therapist. Voice rehabilitation techniques include esophageal speech, voice prosthesis insertion (e.g. Provox or Blom-Singer prosthesis, which is termed neoglottis procedure), or by using a battery-operated artificial larynx, e.g. servox.

107. a. There appears to be right vocal cord immobility most likely resulted from longstanding vocal cord palsy complicating her previous thyroid surgery. Bowing of the affected vocal cord and foreshortening of ipsilateral arytenoid can be observed. There is a significant phonatory gap noted between the vocal cords upon adduction giving clue to a more severe degree of dysphonia (very breathy voice quality) as experienced by this patient. No other significant pathology noted. Thus, the diagnosis is right vocal cord palsy in paramedian position.

b. Certain operative techniques can be performed to bring the paralyzed right vocal cord closer to the functioning contralateral side to improve voice and prevent aspiration (if any).

The ideal final aim is to have an even adduction of the entire membranous vocal cord with restoration of normal mucosal waves upon phonation. These procedure ranges from endoscopic injection [e.g. using fat or calcium hydroxylapatite (CaHA)] to increase the bulk of the paralyzed vocal cord, to open thyroplasty technique with appropriate material inserted (e.g. carved silicone block, Gore-Tex, etc.) to push the paralyzed vocal cord medially. In this patient, thyroplasty technique with or without arytenoid adduction seems appropriate since the gap is moderately large.

108. a. There is a smooth cystic swelling (with straw-colored content) arising from the left membranous vocal cord. The contralateral vocal cord appears thickened like a sessile polyp.

b. Left vocal cord cyst with reactive right vocal cord lesions (likely thickening and polypoid reaction) resulting from chronic collisions caused by the cyst during phonation.

c. The cyst need to be excised/enucleated by using microsurgical technique. The reactive lesion can be left alone initially and postoperatively monitored as it may regress spontaneously; failing which, it can also be excised with prior palpation intraoperatively using special probe for confirmation of fibrosis. However, single session microsurgical intervention for both lesions is being advocated by some with excellent results. Postoperative speech therapy is essential. Small risk of cyst recurrence exists if its wall is incompletely removed.

109. a. Image showed an irregular white lesion along the free edge of left vocal cord extending from the vocal process of arytenoid posteriorly and encroaching toward the anterior commissure.

b. This is very likely to be a leukoplakia. Social history of chronic smoking would raise high suspicion of dysplasia or even malignancy.

c. The examination should proceed further to telescopic assessment of the anterior commissure and subglottic area usually using a 30° or 70° endoscope. Adequate tissue biopsy needs to be taken for histopathological examination. If the report comes back as dysplasia, repeated biopsy needs to be done at another setting determined at follow-up sessions. Subepithelial cordectomy can be performed if there is no evidence of malignancy found. However, if the basement membrane invasion is proved, then the patient needs to be treated as having an invasive carcinoma. In case of clear-cut malignancy, a definitive treatment should be started (usually radiotherapy, this is a T1 lesion with a very favorable prognosis). Alternatively, laser surgery can be performed with equally good result by a formally trained and experienced surgeon.

110. a. Direct laryngoscopy reveals normal vocal cords with narrowing of the subglottic region. The patency of the airway is markedly reduced, which explains the presentation of stridor. The sagittal computed tomography (CT) scan slice shows a tracheostomy *in situ* with a shelf-like stenosis below the vocal cords and above the tracheal stoma.

b. This is a typical finding in subglottic stenosis, which can be acquired (complication of prolonged intubation).

c. Management consists of securing the compromised airway as the very first step. Thereafter, imaging studies are performed (CT scan or magnetic resonance imaging) to delineate the location and thickness of the stenotic component. A thin fibrous stenosis can be excised with laser, while a much thicker one may require a more aggressive surgical treatment ranging from excision to cricoid expansion with costal cartilage or even cricotracheal resection with reanastomosis. In this child, the recommended initial treatment is likely Carbon dioxide (CO_2) laser excision followed by dilatation procedures. Topical mitomycin C application can be considered. Open surgery is advised, when this method fails.

111. a. The vocal cord appears to be of normal appearance and mobility; however, the arytenoids appear to be swollen and edematous. This typically presents as a sensation of foreign body upon swallowing or throat discomfort.

b. This is most likely to be due to laryngopharyngeal reflux (LPR) disease.

c. After a thorough examination of the nose and nasopharynx to rule out chronic rhinosinusitis and postnasal drip, a course of proton pump inhibitors can be prescribed. As inflammation caused by acid reflux heals slowly, a longer course is usually given ranging from 3 weeks to 3 months. Ideally, esophageal pH monitoring should be performed in all cases. However, many laryngologists decided to treat LPR based on symptoms (reflux symptom index) and the typical endoscopic findings. *Helicobaiter pylori* and malignancy should not be missed.

112. This image shows a normal left vocal cord, while the right cord shows a swelling in its mid-membranous portion with an abnormal vessel traversing it and areas of punctate hemorrhage. The abnormal vessel is believed to be involved in the pathogenesis of benign vocal fold lesions including vocal fold cyst and polyp. The normal vocal fold vessels are much finer and run parallel to the long axis of the vocal fold instead of transversely and tortuously, as seen in this image. Bleeding may occur spontaneously or upon voice overuse and it appears as punctate or subepithelial hemorrhage. Repeated events predispose to prolonged reparative changes within the lamina propria layer of the affected vocal cord. Initially, videostroboscopy shows disturbance of mucosal waves, whilst longstanding untreated lesions may manifest itself as polyp, cyst or even Reinke's edema. In addition to the removal of the cyst, this abnormal vessel needs to be ablated usually using a bipolar diathermy at low power setting or alternatively by using laser [usually potassium-titanyl-phosphate laser, or CO_2 laser at defocus mode]. Pulsed dye laser is an excellent alternative for this purpose if available.

113. a. Figure shows symmetric and bilateral nodular whitish swelling affecting the free edge of the true vocal folds at its mid-membranous segment.

b. This appearance is typical of mature vocal fold nodules.
c. Management has to take into account the child's behavior, parent's expectation, peer influence, and the rate of voice recovery to normal. Speech therapy should be the primary treatment in managing pediatric vocal fold nodules and other benign vocal fold lesions. Adequate time and encouragement should be given with the frequency and intensity of voice rehabilitation determined by the speech therapist as the treatment progresses.
d. Surgical excision is needed as the callus appeared well-formed and thickened. Intraoperative palpation gives further information on its consistency. Microsurgical technique is preferred to minimize disturbance of uninvolved areas of the vocal folds.

114. a. There is a yellowish rounded swelling involving the membranous left vocal fold with the fold edge appearing evenly bulging medially. The right vocal fold appeared edematous and its surface whitish in color. The capillary appeared dilated and running parallel along the right vocal fold.
b. Left vocal fold cyst with contralateral reactive vocal fold lesion (likely to be early Reinke's edema with superficial keratoses).
c. Speech therapy is unlikely to resolve the problem, but it should be targeted at postoperative period for optimal healing environment while preventing unsupervised vocal use. She should not be teaching too soon also. Generally, the prognosis of superficial cyst is favorable and unlikely to recur if completely removed (enucleated).
d. Microsurgical excision need to be performed followed by postoperative voice therapy.

115. a. Figure shows the laryngeal inlet view of larynx with visible endotracheal tube. The false vocal folds appeared normal. However, the true vocal folds were obviously swollen and glistening with yellowish tinge seen peripherally.
b. This is typical of Reinke's edema or polypoid corditis. In this condition, there is an accumulation of gelatinous substance like a "gel" in the subepithelial layer or Reinke's space. It commonly occurs in chronic heavy smokers and worsens the voice quality tremendously.
c. Endolaryngeal microsurgery by using cold instruments is generally advocated. A more laterally placed linear incision (cordotomy) can be done by using sickle knife or CO_2 laser. Gelatinous material is then sucked adequately and the epithelium redraped with the excess trimmed. Tissue glue can be applied at the end, but usually it is not necessary.
d. Adequate speech voice rest and speech therapy sessions need to be followed. The patient must quit smoking indefinitely.

116. a. Figure shows injection thyroplasty technique by using autologous fat obtained from the abdominal wall.

b. i. No body rejection
   ii. Abundant material and technically not difficult to harvest
   iii. Direct injection visible under endoscopic view.

c. i. Over injection may cause glottic obstruction and stridor.
   ii. Fat resorption overtime and less than optimal vocal fold approximation.

d. Handheld liposucker for fat aspiration and Bruening syringe for delivery of fat into vocal fold tissue. Presently, several types of high pressure injectors are available to be used for fat injection.

117. a. Figure shows symmetrical reddish swelling located posteriorly beside the endotracheal tube corresponding to the cartilaginous portion of the vocal folds. The false vocal fold and the rest of the true vocal folds appeared normal.

b. This is most likely due to vocal process granuloma or intubation granuloma, a misnomer, if related to previous endotracheal intubation. Too large an endotracheal tube, inadequate sedation, frequent frictions from insecure tube anchoring, prolonged intubation, infections, and LPR disease are amongst the common risk factors implicated for its formation.

c. i. Glottic obstruction due to enlarging granuloma. Stridor can occur upon extubation with variable dysphonia.
   ii. Recurrence after excision. Prophylactic proton pump inhibitor is usually indicated by most laryngologist.

118. a. Figure shows a significant swelling at the tongue base-epiglottis junction or so-called vallecula area. It appears cystic and tense with some linear capillaries seen traversing its surface.

b. Vallecula cyst, which is congenital in this case.

c. Uncapping of the cyst is the most likely procedure, which must be done because much cyst wall together with its covering epithelium, along the perimeter of the cyst needs to be removed. Re-epithelialization from the surrounding normal mucosa will occur upon healing. Initial aspiration allows fluid to be sent for culture and sensitivity as well as making tissue handling during surgery easier.

119. a. These figures show a small upper midline swelling in a child which moves upward upon tongue protrusion.

b. Thyroglossal cyst.

c. Surgical excision is advised as there is a potential risk of recurrence and infection if treated conservatively. The middle part of the hyoid bone is removed together with the cyst, also known as Sistrunk's operation.

120. a. These are the images of Barium Swallow study which shows contrast material along the trachea and lower bronchopulmonary segments bilaterally.

b. This is diagnostic of barium aspiration.

c. Barium causes inflammatory response along the tracheobronchial mucosa and pneumonitis. It takes sometimes for the contrast to disappear naturally but the lung functions need to be monitored closely if significant aspiration like this one happened. Ward admission, parenteral corticosteroid and antibiotic cover are administered. Oxygen saturation (SaO_2) monitoring and blood gases are taken, with oxygen delivered whenever indicated.

121. a. There is bright red appearance affecting the dorsal aspect of the right true vocal fold beneath its epithelium. This finding is typical of acute subepithelial hemorrhage which occurs upon voice overuse. There are no other benign lesions or LPR changes seen.

b. She needs to rest the voice completely over the next 3–5 days and thereafter may resume phonation gradually as advised by the speech language pathologist. She should refrain herself from singing back too early to allow for normal healing to take place naturally. Repeated hemorrhage may cause scar changes and permanent dysphonia if not addressed correctly. The laryngologist will reassess the vocal fold and look out possible treatable cause such as vascular ectasia and varix.

122. These are two types of endotracheal tubes used for the purpose of microlaryngeal surgery. The metallic tube is malleable (flexometallic) and has two cuffs at its distal end which are filled with colored saline. The other is normal endotracheal tube with single distal cuff and was wrapped proximally with shiny reflective tape to conceal the actual tube.

These are the suitable tubes and their modifications intended to be used for laser microlaryngeal surgery. They prevent the laser beam striking and puncturing into the endotracheal lumen which can cause explosion and airway fire. The double cuff offer additional protection as the more distal cuff can still seal the endotracheal wall if the more proximal cuff burst.

123. a. These are the endoscopic laryngeal images showing a bluish swelling with nodular surface alike to mulberry fruit involving the right supraglottic larynx and encroaching the medial aspect of ipsilateral pyriform fossa. The appearance suggests a vascular tumor most likely hemangioma. Depending on patient's symptoms and rate of growth, the possibility of malignant transformations need to be considered. General examination should rule out similar lesions elsewhere.

b. Magnetic resonance imaging with contrast would delineate the extent and vascularity of the tumor especially in an attempt to identify the blood vessels feeders amenable for embolization if this is decided to be done.

c. In experienced hand, this can be excised surgically via transoral approach. Good homeostatic device must be available, e.g. suction diathermy or insulated bipolar diathermy and the used of suitable laser, e.g. Nd:Yag or pulsed dye laser. An alternative is via lateral pharyngotomy approach.

124. a. The first figure reveals an end-tracheostomy with a voice prosthesis *in situ* (Blom-Singer) while the other shows an endoscopic view of the pharyngoesophageal segment upon phonation by using the prosthesis.

b. This is a form of voice rehabilitation to enable phonation after total laryngectomy. The voice prosthesis gives a better and clearer voice as compared to oesophageal voice and can be learned faster. Occlusion of the end-tracheostomy is necessary to shunt the exhaled air into the pharyngoesophageal segment. However, innovation and current technology has made hands-free technique possible, which gives great freedom and boosts the patient's morale tremendously.